Also by Elaine LaLanne:
FITNESS AFTER 50

DYNASTRIDE! (SM)

Elaine LaLanne's
Complete Walking Program
for Fitness After 50

DYNASTRIDE! _(SM)

Elaine LaLanne's
Complete Walking Program
for Fitness After 50
with Richard Benyo

THE STEPHEN GREENE PRESS
Lexington, Massachusetts

ACKNOWLEDGEMENTS

I'm grateful to: Richard Benyo, for his concepts and collabora-
tions; doctors Yvonne LaLanne, D.C., Mark Rubenstein, M.D.,
Omar Fareed, M.D., John C. Schwarting, D.C., and Gail Shem-
well, Ph.D., nutritionist, for their advice; Liz Cardenas, my
assistant, who is often both my right and left hand; Rhonda
Provost, Catherine Solicito, Kevin Kerslake, Hattie Montez, and
Uncle Bernard Rorem; all the wise LaLanneisms by which I try
to live; and Tom Begner, my publisher, who made it all happen.

Copyright © Specific Publications, Inc., 1988
All rights reserved

First published in 1988 by The Stephen Greene Press, Inc.
Published simultaneously in Canada by Penguin Books Canada Limited
Distributed by Viking Penguin Inc., 40 West 23rd Street, New York,
NY 10010.

Photographs by Kevin Kerslake.
Line drawings by Susan Levine.

Dynastride℠ is a service mark of Befit Enterprises.

Library of Congress Cataloging-in-Publication Data

LaLanne, Elaine
  Dynastride! : Elaine LaLanne's walking program for
fitness after 50.

  1. Physical fitness.   2. Walking.   I. Title.
GV481.L29 1988   613.7'1   87-21118
ISBN 0-8289-0632-7

Printed in the United States of America
by The Alpine Press

Set in Palatino

DEDICATION:

To my sons,
Dan and Jon,
who are so supportive
of everything I do;
to Dr. Yvonne,
who has lived through my second
book and given me her input: I
couldn't ask for a more
wonderful daughter;
and to my daughter,
Janet,
in Heaven.
Again,
to my husband,
Jack:
Without you I couldn't
have written either
book . . . I love you!

Contents

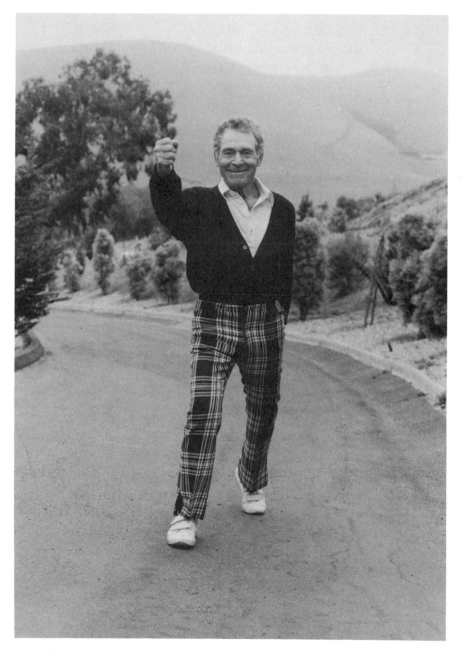

The Original Dynastrider—Jack devised the concept of Dynastriding℠ 50 years ago, and I have integrated it as an essential part of my walking programs.

Foreword: What Is Dynastriding ⓈⓂ?

When most people walk, they seldom use their arms. Your arms perform an important function for your body, and by using them properly, you can improve your posture, firm up the shoulders and chest, and give yourself greater cardiovascular conditioning.

This is where Dynastriding comes in. Dynastriding merely means that instead of taking regular (easy) strides, the length of each stride is increased so it is not only taxing the leg, hip and back muscles, but also the ligaments, tendons, and joints. This not only helps make them more flexible and youthful, but also provides a greater range of motion.

So, when you Dynastride, exaggerate standing tall, draw in your waist as tightly as you can, swing your arms in motion with your legs and, as you stride out, swing your arms back and forward (even over your head as far as they'll go). The combination of using your big leg and back muscles while walking, and the dozens of other muscles that are used while swinging your arms, gives you double benefit from your walking program.

Let me tell you about how I came up with Dynastriding.

It has always been my feeling that we have had the gift of walking since we were approximately one year old.

We improved upon this ability throughout our childhood, and refined it even more in adulthood. Then, at the moment we had the ability to walk at its height, many of us began to deteriorate. (Only a small portion of the population became athletes or went into some sort of physical activity.) There are several reasons for the fact that most adults began to decline. The number one reason is we learned to drive a car or had someone drive us to our destination. But it didn't stop there. We also rode in airplanes, in elevators, on escalators, in golf carts. When people ride too much it takes away the ability to walk well and, as we grow older, certain changes sometimes occur to us that walking could have prevented: arthritis, rheumatism, heart problems and other aches and pains.

Walking is a gift we should discover again because if walking is done correctly, it works so many muscles in the body.

I started thinking seriously about walking shortly after I opened the first modern physical culture studio in 1936. What started me thinking about walking was meeting a gentleman by the name of Bernar MacFadden, who started one of the first physical culture magazines. (Bernar Mac-Fadden later owned his own publishing company and became a millionaire.) He was considered a health nut—a real nature boy, with long hair and sandals.

He became famous not only by spending large amounts of money trying to become President of the United States, but by leading large groups of people on long walks in parks, around ocean beach areas, and in the mountains.

Back in those days, walking to me meant the act of strolling. And strolling wasn't my idea of exercise. Another thing that bothered me about walking was that we had been casually walking all our lives and any exercise, in order to be beneficial, had to become progressively more vigorous. You see, the muscles only respond if they are challenged beyond what they are used to doing. Bernar MacFadden proved to me that people were interested in walking, and I wanted to help them get more exercise while they were doing it.

I had already devised a plan of progressive weight training and stretching (done aerobically) for my students. Now I felt it was time to devise a plan of progressive walking. I called this plan "dynamic walking" or Dynastriding.

I should mention that stretching is very important, too, especially when you reach your 40s, 50s and 60s. Lack of vigorous exercise can cause ligaments and tendons to become stiff and unyielding. However, you can improve elasticity in these important areas by stretching them regularly.

I'm really excited about Elaine's walking book! She is as conscientious and enthusiastic as I am about physical fitness and wants to get every man, woman and child eating and exercising properly. There is a tremendous need for this book because there are so many Americans, young and old, who are just not getting enough exercise.

Although Elaine is in her 60s, she has the body of a 30-year-old and is a true example of what exercise and proper nutrition can do for you. I'm positive that what she has to offer on the following pages will not only help you, but many thousands of people, to get off their seat and onto their feet.

—Jack LaLanne

Introduction
You Can Walk Your Way To Good Health

"Henry Ford got the people off their feet and onto the seat. I want to get them off their seat and onto their feet."
—Jack LaLanne, 1952
KGO-TV, San Francisco

The first time I heard the "LaLannism" of "I want to get the people off their seat and onto their feet," I thought to myself, "Oh, isn't that cute?" and let it go at that.

At the time I was working at KGO-TV in San Francisco on the Les Malloy daily variety show. The show was on from 4:30 to 6:30 each weekday afternoon. The format was very similar to today's talk shows. I was called a Girl Friday. Today I would be called a co-host. Among the things I was responsible for was booking guests for the show. I suppose you could say I was Ed McMahon to Les Malloy's Johnny Carson.

Like most people involved in a day-in-day-out job, I had settled into a sort of rut that included lots of pressure, no exercise, and plenty of junk food. In fact, I hadn't exercised in eight years and my daily intake included cigarettes, coffee, chocolate donuts, Danish bear claws, candy bars, and ice cream. A real junk food junkie. Then one day, POW!!! A human dynamo popped into my life: Jack LaLanne. He began a daily morning exercise program on the station and got me off my seat and onto my feet.

I related most of the story of how I met Jack in my first book, *Fitness After 50,* but one story I didn't include in that book is how I started my walking routine.

One day Jack asked me if I liked to hike. I immediately said, "Yes." I was remembering eight or nine years before when I had done a lot of hiking and had taken long walks in the woods back in Minnesota. Well, Jack invited me to join him for a hike up the ledge trail in Yosemite National Park in

California. At that time I had never been to Yosemite but I thought I was coming prepared for this hike. Little did I know—

This hike was straight up the side of a mountain. One mile almost straight up. I started out just fine, but then the trail became steeper and steeper. With his tremendous endurance, Jack was moving right along while I was trying desperately to keep up with him. Believe me, I was getting mighty tired quickly and was suffering from that disease Jack was always talking about on his show: Pooped-Out-Itis.

I finally had to give in and admit how tired I was. Jack proved once again to be Jack. He told me to climb up on his back and he'd carry me for a while. Even being carried, I was huffing and puffing, thirsty as a racehorse and sorry that I had ever heard the word "hike," when we came upon a mountain stream gurgling with clear, fresh water.

I literally jumped into the stream, lay flat on my stomach, and lapped up the water like a thirsty dog. I wanted only one more thing at that point: to give up. I wanted to go back down the mountain. "I can't go on," I moaned from the stream.

Jack told me to rest for a few minutes, and as we did, he offered me help and encouragement. We started out again, and went a little farther. Every step we moved upward, I repeated to myself, "Never again. Never again."

We eventually made it to the top. What an introduction to a walking program! I think it's pretty clear that I'd gone about it the wrong way.

If I knew then what I know now, I wouldn't have even started that hike. But it was a lesson learned. I didn't tell Jack that I hadn't exercised in many years because I wasn't aware that eight years could make such a change in my physical condition. He was always saying on his show, "Make haste slowly." I had received a dramatic lesson in what happens if you don't follow that philosophy.

Most people—unfortunately—do not have Jack there to help them along. Even with Jack's help, though, I learned that ultimately we have to carry ourselves no matter what we do. *We, and we alone, are responsible for our lives.* We must be honest with ourselves and learn to like and love ourselves. I don't mean in an egotistical way, but in a way that will benefit society and ultimately get the best for ourselves out of our individual lives. Our attitude is what counts. If we say, "I can't!" we'll quickly find out that we were right: we can't.

Generally, I'm a positive person. However, I'm not a stranger to the "I can't" syndrome.

In my freshman year at the University of Minnesota, I remember coming home and sitting on the steps leading upstairs. I was talking with my father. "I'm no good," I told him. "I'm not talented, I don't know where I'm going in life. I don't seem to have any goals. I can't seem to get my life together and I feel inferior." I genuinely felt that way. I believed what I was saying. No doubt many of you have felt the same way at times.

My father was quite an armchair philosopher and we often spent many hours together talking about life and living. He always said, "There are two sides to every story." But he also left the decisions up to me. In the course of our conversation, he said, "You were vice-president of your senior class, you were a cheerleader, you were on the student council." Then he said: "You learned to swim, didn't you?"

His reference to my swimming really hit me, because I had found it very difficult to learn to swim, especially learning to ballet swim. I eventually swam in the Minneapolis Aqua Follies and to me, this was a big accomplishment.

My father's statement helped reinforce my confidence and made me realize that I was capable of doing anything to which I set my mind. You see, the other accomplishments he had mentioned had come somewhat easy to me. But the swimming—that was different. I had had to learn to swim at the same time I was attempting to overcome the fear that I could not do it. I don't know which was worse.

You may fear that you don't have the ability to stay on a diet to lose weight, to attend a community college when you're well past what we consider "college age," to stay on a regular exercise program or to do any number of other things. But remember that fear begets fear and fear begets the "I can't" syndrome.

Even though a regular exercise program and good nutrition did not become a part of my life until I met Jack, I had wrestled often with periods of ups and downs in my life. The memory of the "I can't" syndrome made me worry that even with Jack's help, I would not be able to turn my life around. But I found that the exercise and nutrition program reinforced itself as it went, and had positive effects on everything in my life.

You see, when you are physically fit, you are mentally fit. The more mentally fit you become, the less fear you have. This leads to more confidence in yourself.

If you are sedentary, your blood flow becomes sluggish and you become lethargic. When your blood flow is accelerated by exercise, you become more alert and less sluggish. What better way to activate the blood and eliminate sluggishness than by taking a simple step: walk. Walking is the most basic exercise of all.

Done well, a good, brisk walk in the Dynastriding style can be the most satisfying ingredient of any day. And while it is uplifting, it also bestows many health benefits. In addition to the physical benefits of improving muscles and raising cardiovascular efficiency, walking is a terrific stress reliever. It can create a special time in your day that promotes clear thinking while building a sense of well-being and increased self-esteem. And yes, a regular walking program, done at a prescribed effort, helps burn away unwanted body fat.

All these good results come without pills, surgery or going on fad diets that never work for very long.

In this book, I'll tell you about walking: what it does for your body (and your head) and how it can best be practiced. The book will also present walking-for-health programs that *you* can employ which will help change your life for the better.

So put your best foot forward. I'm going to help you improve your walkability!

—Elaine LaLanne
Morro Bay, California
March 1988

PART I

Walking Is For Everyone

Chapter 1

Why Should I Walk?

"Walking is man's best medicine."

—Hippocrates

Has it ever occurred to you that the human being is one of the only creatures on earth that occupies every continent? The reason people have spread to virtually every spot on the earth is because they are both mobile and adaptable, and that mobility has always come from the legs.

These early humans used their strong legs to run down game. By making use of an alternating walk/jog, human hunters ran their game, often larger than themselves, to exhaustion, tiring the game until it was too weak to resist. Result: Food to exist. When the game supply ran out in one area, the hunters used those well-developed leg muscles to hike off to the next horizon to satisfy their need for food and their curiosity to discover what was over the next mountain.

Between following food sources and satisfying curiosity, we human beings eventually ended up in every nook and cranny on earth, propelled there by legs that were made for walking.

Although it is such a marvelous—and functional—part of the human anatomy, the human leg is really a simple piece of machinery. (The ankle and foot are much more complex.)

There are only four bones in each human leg. The largest bone in the leg (and in the body) is the femur, which is the bone between the hip and the knee and is the only bone in the thigh. The lower leg has two bones, the tibia (or shin bone) and the

much smaller fibula, which is just beside the tibia and on the outside of the leg.

The fourth bone is the kneecap, called the patella.

The ends of the bones are covered with cartilage and held together by ligaments. Very simple construction, but very effective. Of course, if all we had were bones, the leg would be completely immobile. And, when the first wind came along, the human skeleton would be blown over.

The bones are given their mobility, and the legs their strength, by carefully placed muscles. Think of the bones as the framework over which the muscles are stretched. The legs not only contain the largest bones in the body, but also the largest muscles: large muscles to move large bones. Sit in a chair and let's become familiar with the leg muscles. There aren't many to learn, so don't feel overwhelmed. The leg muscles are so large that there isn't really any need for a great number of them.

While seated, place your right palm on the lower end of your right thigh, just behind the knee. Spread your fingers. Now, hold your thigh steady (parallel to the floor) and extend your leg. Feel the muscles tensing and bunching under your fingers? The big muscles that make up the front of the thigh are the quadriceps, and their companion muscle (the longest muscle in the body) is called the sartorius. Now, slide your hand to the inside of

1

your thigh and feel the adductor muscle by moving your thigh to the right and to the left. At the rear of the thigh (the underside if you're still sitting) is the biceps femoris (hamstring). Reach behind your leg and grab the big hamstring. The hamstring returns the leg to its original position.

On the lower leg, it's much the same but reversed. The big muscles are in the back: the gastrocnemius and the soleus form the calf, the muscle group in the body with the most densely packed muscle fibers. Your calf is the heart of your lymphatic system. It acts upon your lymphatic system as your heart acts upon your vascular system.

Now, wasn't that easy? Each leg has only four bones, and both the upper leg (thigh) and the lower leg (the shin) each have four, simple muscle groups. The legs are supplied with blood by the longest arteries in the body, as those big muscles need plenty of oxygen- and nutrient-carrying blood in order to "do their thing."

Because the leg muscles are the largest in the body, any exercise that works the legs will effectively make the cardiovascular system (heart, lungs, and the blood vessels) perform more effectively. This work promotes fitness. The most important kind of fitness you can develop is cardiovascular fitness. One way to do this is through the regular use of the leg muscles in a repetitive manner, such as walking.

Walking is the use to which the human leg is best suited, because it is the major exercise humans have been doing well for the longest period of time—ever since the first human being took the first upright step.

Health Benefits

What is the meaning of the word *health*?

The dictionary gives this definition: "That state of being in which all parts and organs are sound and in proper condition." My interpretation: I believe that health is the presence of strong, vital body signs indicating that a person is taking an active role in his or her own physical well-being.

A regular walking program, even if it is taken up later in life, can help improve these health-regulating systems and conditions:

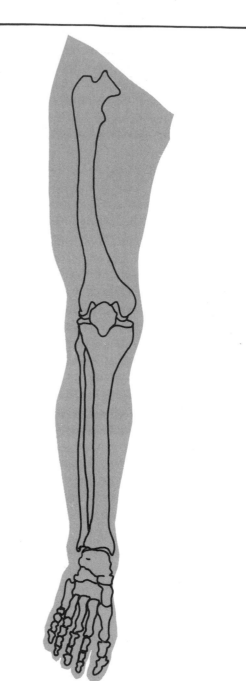

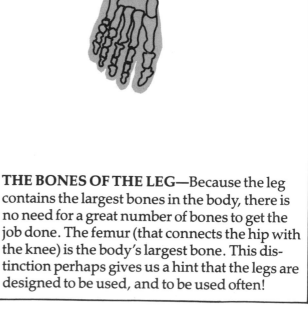

THE BONES OF THE LEG—Because the leg contains the largest bones in the body, there is no need for a great number of bones to get the job done. The femur (that connects the hip with the knee) is the body's largest bone. This distinction perhaps gives us a hint that the legs are designed to be used, and to be used often!

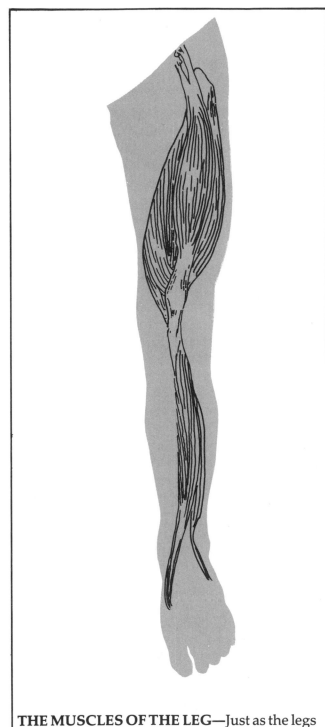

THE MUSCLES OF THE LEG—Just as the legs feature the body's largest bones, they can also brag about containing the largest muscles and the most densely-packed muscle groups. The quadriceps and the biceps femoris (the muscles in the front and back of the thigh) are huge compared to other muscles in the body. Any use of these huge muscles translates into high calorie use.

1. **Blood Pressure**. One of the major signs that tells us our body is not working well and is in deep trouble is high blood pressure. High blood pressure is both an indication that something has gone wrong and that they are in immediate need of correction. A regular, modest but vigorous walking program will help lower blood pressure, depending on the cause. And that's a very positive step toward good health.

2. **Body Fat**. There are very few of us who are not concerned, to some extent, with excessive body fat. Most of us just simply have too much body fat. With the fat comes unwanted weight, sagging in places, bloating in other places, premature aging, deterioration of body organs and parts, and a general feeling of frustration. Excess fat can also promote diseases of the heart, diabetes, etc. Any regular aerobic style exercise will help burn calories. Calories are stored in fatty tissue (roughly 3500 calories equal one pound of body fat), and with exercise these stored calories are burned to provide energy. As more calories are burned, body fat drops. Slow, repetitive aerobic exercise burns fat calories best. However, what you put into your mouth also plays an important role in determining your fat content.

3. **Cholesterol**. Cholesterol is a major contributor to cardiovascular disease. It forms plaque on the insides of the arteries, and over the years this build-up of plaque narrows down the passageways, restricting the flow of blood. If the arteries are blocked, ultimately, the heart (no matter how strong it is) becomes suffocated because the oxygen and nutrients it needs to keep functioning are not reaching it fast enough. Throw in a situation where the body is under stress (a sickness or an emergency situation that calls for quick physical action), and you've got a heart attack. Brisk walking (an aerobic exercise) done regularly helps cut down cholesterol. Walking, as in an exercise program, should be coupled with a careful diet low in cholesterol.

4. **Resting Pulse Rate**. Your resting pulse rate (the number of times per minute your heart beats while you are at rest) is an indicator of just how efficiently your heart is working. The lower the pulse rate, the more efficiently the heart is functioning. Count your resting pulse rate first thing in the morning before you get out of bed. A 50 to 90

resting pulse rate is considered normal. Regular, aerobic exercise brings the pulse rate down as it makes the heart perform more efficiently. (We'll get into resting pulse rate more thoroughly in Chapter 5.)

5. **Metabolism**. As we grow older, our metabolic rate slows. Metabolism is the rate at which our bodies burn fuel (food and stored fat) in order to operate essential body systems and to maintain and repair those systems. When you were 16, your metabolism was very, very high because your body was growing at an incredible rate and it had tremendous energy needs. When the growth period ended, and especially as you grew older, the metabolic rate slowed and was directed only toward repairing and maintaining body systems.

Unfortunately, we often continue to eat as though we were 16. Or, we cut back on our food intake but not at the rate we should—certainly not as quickly as our metabolism slows. *And*, we became less active physically. One solution is to speed up our metabolism again by regular exercise.

6. **Sleep**. A regular exercise program promotes restorative, refreshing sleep.

7. **Regularity**. Irregularity of bowel movements is a product of poor eating habits and a sedentary lifestyle. Regularity often decreases as we age. This deterioration of function is said to be three times as common among women as men. It is a very uncomfortable fact of life for many people and constipation can jeopardize one's health.

A vigorous walking program and good nutrition (including attention to fiber intake) helps promote regularity.

8. **Healthy Heart**. One of the most frequent causes of death in America is heart disease. Heart disease usually takes one of two forms: either the arteries become clogged and literally suffocate the heart (see #3 above), or the heart muscle itself becomes flabby, weak, and therefore inefficient as a pump, often in conjunction with the first.

A dynamic, regular walking program helps strengthen the heart muscle and promotes healthy, functioning arteries. And, wonderfully enough, this improvement in the heart and the vascular system begins happening within weeks of taking up a regular walking program!

Fitness Benefits

I recently asked Jack, "What are the benefits of being fit?" He answered simply, "To feel good and to look good."

The dictionary defines a fit person as "someone in good health or in good physical condition." The *World Book* goes into great detail, but in general it says that there is a close relationship between a person's health and physical fitness; that muscular activity aids bodily functions.

Many people think that fitness means running marathon races, competing in triathlons, or performing some kind of incredible feat, such as Jack did on his 70th birthday: towing 70 people in 70 rowboats while handcuffed and with feet shackled for a distance of one and one-half miles in Long Beach Harbor near the Queen Mary. People who take on these personal challenges want not only to become physically fit but to reach a certain level of performance in their particular field. However, for the average person it doesn't take that kind of exercise to be physically fit. The key word is consistency. Develop a healthy lifestyle!

Many people, especially those over 50, also think that aerobic fitness means running and jumping for an hour to music. Therefore, they literally give up doing anything physical because it is too difficult for them. They don't realize that aerobic fitness means bringing oxygen into the blood stream by doing something physical (such as brisk walking: Dynastriding) for a sustained period of time (at least 15 minutes). As the heart rate increases, more oxygen-carrying blood is pumped through the body to help burn off stored fat.

Our bodies can store food but not oxygen. If you are in good physical condition, the oxygen helps burn up the stored food and produce energy. In the poorly conditioned body, it is hard for the oxygen when drawn into the lungs to get to those places where the food is stored. This situation produces a tired feeling, or that disease called Pooped-Out-Itis (a Jack LaLannism).

Now let's take a moment to look at several areas of fitness that Dynastriding affects:

1. **Cardiovascular Effectiveness**. Brisk walking or Dynastriding (striding out by making active use

of the arms) helps improve cardiovascular efficiency. Why? Because you are using the big muscle groups; for example, the legs, buttocks, and lower back. All these muscles are working simultaneously, helping to pass along the oxygen and nutrients through the bloodstream, thus helping to produce energy.

2. **Muscle Tone**. The human body has over 600 muscles. These muscles make it possible for us to perform the many functions of which we are capable. Muscles make the heart beat, blood circulate, and help pass the food through the digestive tract. So when you don't use these muscles they become weak and flabby; they start to atrophy and lose their tone. Regular exercise and walking done briskly promote good muscle tone.

3. **Strength**. Strength is energy. The more active you are, the more strength you will have. It's like putting money in the bank. The more you put in, the more you can take out. Therefore, if you are inactive, your body becomes sedentary and physically bankrupt.

4. **Flexibility**. Everyone, regardless of age, can improve flexibility. Muscles are fastened to the bones by ligaments, which are like cords or bands. In fact, think of them as rubber bands. If those rubber bands do not get stretched, they lose their flexibility and become brittle. The same is true with tendons and muscles. If they don't get used or stretched, they become stiff and inflexible. It's a matter of the old saying of "Use it or lose it." If you don't use your muscles, ligaments, and tendons, you're going to lose the benefit of their usefulness.

5. **Increased Ability To Do Other Work**. The human body is the only machine ever produced that gets better the more it is used. By regularly exercising, the body is taught to move more efficiently and with more strength and endurance. This improved capacity carries over into every aspect of one's life. A fit body is a happy body.

Psychological Benefits

I believe that you can't separate the mind from the body. To help prove my point, try this experiment with me. Pretend you don't have a worry in the world, that everything in your life is going fantastically: plenty of money, a brand new car, children all perfect, etc. Now, take your right hand and pull back the middle finger of your left hand as far as possible. Painful, isn't it? Are you thinking of your perfect life right now? No, you are thinking about the pain. When we are in pain or not feeling well, we are not in the best of spirits and the world around us is pretty bleak. However, if we are feeling well and our spirits are up, we feel that we can handle anything that comes along. Our entire outlook changes.

The President's Council on Physical Fitness and Sports has statistics that tell us that many of our aches and pains come from lack of physical activity. Many of us have those little aches and pains which make us less efficient. So let's make it our goal to rid ourselves of those little irritants. And what better way than to start from the beginning with something we've been doing all our lives: walking.

A regular walking program, with its fitness benefits, also brings with it a variety of psychological benefits:

1. **Peace of Mind**. Equanimity. It means evenness of mind, composure, peace of mind. Equanimity comes from feeling good, and when you *feel* good you also *look* good, which in turn makes you feel even better. So, with good health on your side, due to a regular walking program, you can attain that state of being which is blissful. If we wish to participate and promote equanimity, it's within our reach.

2. **Problem Solving**. A psychologist friend of mine has been telling me for years that it isn't the big problems that bring a person down, but rather the accumulation of the smaller ones. Those little, nagging problems pile up before you know it and their accumulated weight can bring you down. I like to think of problems as experiences. Often, when I am Dynastriding down the road, I find these little experiences that I have found hard to solve . . . solved! How? One way is letting go. Sometimes, we are so up-tight we can't see the forest for the trees, but when we become relaxed by striding through the trees, we can let go so our minds can figure out a solution.

3. **Stress Relief**. How do you spell relief? I'll tell

you. Haven't you had one or two of those incredibly stressful days when your neck and shoulders were tight and painful? Chronic headaches are also a manifestation of stress. What is your solution? A pill? Or do you have some other answer? Let me ask you, If you had a nail in your shoe and it was very painful to walk, would you take a pill or would you pull out the nail? Simple. Find the cause and pull out the nail, of course. It's a matter of cause and effect. Often we treat the effect but never stop to consider the cause. The cause for those tensions and stresses which sometimes produce pain could be due to lack of physical activity. Tension has often triggered severe pain in my neck and shoulders, particularly since having been hit from behind when a bus lost its brakes and smashed into the rear end of my car. If it hadn't been for a regular exercise program, not only would I have been more severely injured, but I'm sure I wouldn't be in as good shape as I'm in today. However, consistency is the secret. I find that, when I am not consistent with my exercising, the old aches and pains come back. Physical activity is a tension reliever and a wonderful therapy for stress. If we no longer perceive a situation as being stressful, it will cease to *be* stressful.

4. **Self-Esteem**. How is your self-esteem? High or low? I'm sure that you have some friends with high and some with low self-esteem. For the most part, have you noticed that the ones with high self-esteem seem to have a high energy level and the ones with low self-esteem a low energy level? I've noticed that the more physically fit people are, the better they feel about themselves. I've also seen people over 50 who have been minimally physical during their lives begin a regular walking program, and within six months a miracle happens. They have more confidence in themselves, more energy, blood pressure is lowered, and they seem to be more mentally alert. It is as though they have been given a new lease on life. When you feel better physically, you not only look good but you feel better about yourself.

5. **You're In Charge**. Who's in charge here? Who dictates to whom? Does your body dictate to you, or do you dictate to your body? When you say to your body, "Let's go, let's move, let's go for a walk," what does your body say? "I'm too tired, I'm too busy, I'm too old, not today, maybe tomorrow"? It should be the other way around. When you tell your body to move, it should be happy to move to do whatever you ask it to do. The more the body moves, the more it wants to move. Remember the law of physics: a body in motion tends to stay in motion until acted upon by some outside force. So make your first move! Put your best foot forward to walk, and the more you walk, the more you will want to walk.

So, Why Walk?

Considering the health, fitness, and psychological benefits inherent in a regular walking program, the question should not be, "Why should I walk?" It should be rephrased to read: "Why *not* walk?"

Chapter 2

What Kind Of Walking Is Best?

"Exercise has the effect of defusing anger and rage, fear and anxiety. Like music, it soothes the savage in us that lies so close to the surface. It is the ultimate tranquilizer."

—Dr. George Sheehan

What's all this noise about walking, anyway? Isn't walking a simple, basic, long-standing human characteristic? What's so hard about putting one foot in front of the other?

Actually, there's nothing profoundly complicated about walking if it is kept that simple.

But if we are to get something positive out of walking, it must be done with an eye toward getting the most benefit possible.

The object of a walking program for fitness and health, which is the core of the program detailed in this book, is to physically and psychologically benefit not just from the walking, but from the results of a regular walking program.

In the most basic terms, there is a big difference between simply "strolling" and walking for fitness and health.

Walking for fitness and health involves striving for a training effect.

What is a training effect?

You will achieve a training effect when you stress your body to a point beyond that to which it is accustomed.

It means putting greater demands on your muscles and circulatory system. The more the muscles are challenged, the more they respond.

In order to get better at walking, you have to work hard enough to improve your ability to do it.

If you go strolling along a street, stopping to window shop, you are not gaining a training effect from and for walking. You are training for window shopping.

The training effect comes into play when you exercise your heart muscle by making it work harder for the distance of your walk than it would work while watching TV or sleeping or strolling past shop windows.

The fact that you have raised your heart rate and held it there (see Chapter 5) for let's say 20 minutes, trains your heart to function more efficiently at both the increased heart rate and at your normal resting heart rate. Therefore, the next time you walk there will be some training effect present from the previous time. This is because your heart and circulatory system will be able to increase their work at that elevated heart rate induced by your vigorous walking.

The more you walk (as long as you don't overdo it), the more you are actually training your heart to become stronger and more efficient. Your heart will also be more efficient when just sitting around idling, and it will be able to idle at a lower speed rather than at the higher speed it was used to before you started an exercise program.

Take, for instance, your car. If it idles too fast you either take it to a mechanic or fix it yourself to get it to idle slower. Let me explain further.

For example, when you start your program, perhaps your pulse rate (heart beat) will be 90 times a minute when you awake in the morning (the best time to measure your pulse rate). After six months of my walking program, your resting pulse rate upon rising in the morning may be down to 78. What this means is that your heart is doing the same amount of work as before but at 12 beats less per minute. It is becoming more efficient.

If your heart is more efficient, it will respond better when an emergency comes along.

This may lead you to ask: "Just how often do I have to take my heart out for a walk if I want to gain this training effect?"

There can be benefits from doing it three or four times a week. But my own feeling is that the more regular a part of your life you make your walking program, whether you are 15 or 115, the better off you are. Consistency is the key. *As long as you don't overdo it!*

I know that when I'm at home between traveling dates, I like to resume set patterns. It simplifies my life and removes a great deal of stress. My husband, Jack, is the same, even when we are on the road. At home he gets up before the sun and does his workout. On the road he's likely to rearrange the furniture in our hotel room so he can still get up before the sun and do his exercise program before breakfast. We both thrive on that consistency.

Therefore, I advise people to include walking in their *daily* lives. Which means to me doing it four to six times a week, or even seven times a week. You'll see this regularity reflected in my walking programs (Chapters 8, 9, 10 and 11), and I'll be referring to it regularly as we go along.

For any program like this to work, it *must* become as normal to you as getting out of bed in the morning and as regular as brushing your teeth. I believe you eat every day, you sleep every day, your body was made to exercise every day. Once you have made Dynastriding a regular part of your day, its value to you will soar.

I don't want this walking program to be boring,

so we're not going to do the same exercise every day.

My programs offer variety along with consistency. If you walk far or long one day, the next day or two will be relatively easy so that your body will have time to recover from the hard workout so that the training effect will have an opportunity to come into play.

Walking that is done intelligently and vigorously can lead to basic fitness in approximately two months. As you become better conditioned, you are capable of doing more and more and more.

Believe me when I tell you that what seemed like a real challenge near the beginning will seem like less than a warm-up stroll after several months.

Walking has many advantages. Among my favorites are these:

1. You can incorporate your walking program into what you are doing during your normal day. For example, if you have to go to the store, you can work out a course that allows you to take a long route so that you not only get your day's walking in, but do your shopping at the same time. If you live far enough away from the store that walking is impractical, simply drive your car part of the way and walk the rest. If necessary, buy a two-wheel rolling basket.

2. You don't need a radical change of clothes for walking, so you can do it when you want, where you want, without advanced preparation.

3. When you purchase a good pair of walking shoes, you will find that they are the most comfortable shoes you're ever going to own. You'll probably end up wearing them exclusively. You know as well as I do that when your feet hurt, you hurt all over. Good walking shoes can be a balm for the feet.

4. Walking can be done almost anywhere at any time. You can walk in the local park or at the South Pole, in a mall or around the block, on a cruise ship or up the side of a mountain.

5. You can walk alone or with a close friend or with a whole group of people and it is equally beneficial.

6. The more you walk, the more you *can* walk.

7. It is the easiest—and most universal—of all aerobic exercises.

8. There is no age, race, sex, political or religious barrier to it.

The Many Forms of Walking

There is strolling, walking, striding, power-walking, exercise-walking, race-walking, hiking, trekking, and Dynastriding.

For the purposes of my walking program, there are only three types of walking you need to know about, and as soon as we mention them, you can forget about the first one.

The three types are strolling, walking and Dynastriding.

1. . . . **Strolling**. Strolling is the process of meandering more than walking. It is what you do when you window shop: you move slowly and with a seemingly aimless purpose from one store window to the next. It is also what two lovers do in the moonlight. This is not significant aerobic exercise. The only way you'll perspire while strolling is if the temperature is 95 degrees and so is the humidity.

2. . . . **Walking**. This is the process of moving from one location to another by foot at a gentle but purposeful pace. The respiratory rate is not raised to any significant degree. The extent of the exercise involves toning the leg muscles. Additionally, there is the benefit of getting out in the air with your own thoughts. Traditionally this is called taking a daily constitution.

3. . . . **Dynastriding** (vigorous walking). This is walking with vigor, with a purpose, with efficient but energetic use of both arms and legs. The exact pace is not important to our discussion at this point. The positive effects of walking occur at very different speeds depending on the physical

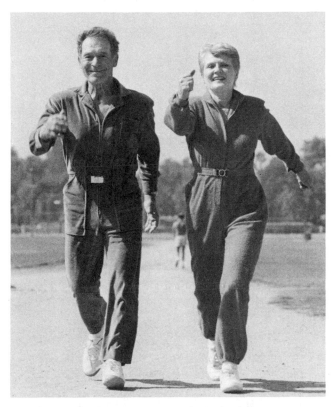 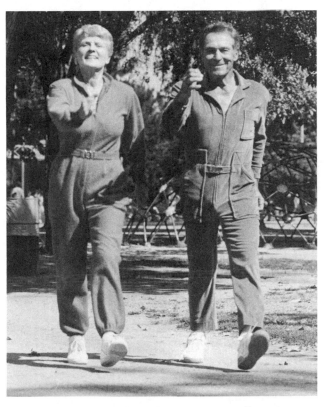

DYNASTRIDE!—In order to get the most out of your walking, you must elevate it to a point where it is making use of the whole body. That is the Dynastriding concept. Make maximum use of the arms and legs, swinging them in rhythm and as far as they will comfortably go. Don't feel that you need to be able to come to full stride as soon as you start your program. Begin conservatively and gradually build until you are able to stride out with vigor and authority. Lift those legs! Swing those arms! Breathe deeply! Walk with vigor and you'll generate more vitality. Learn to make your walking rely upon the entire body!

condition of the person walking. The experienced walker makes this vigorous walking look smooth and effortless even though the body is getting a good workout. This is the type of walking you will be striving for; it is the type of walking that brings the cornucopia of physical and psychological benefits. Once you have achieved this level, it does not mean that you will never again be able to stroll or merely walk. It means, instead, that you have taken the giant step into a whole 'nother kind of walking.

Determining Your Current Level

Although we will thoroughly discuss (in Chapter 5) the process of regulating your walking program according to your pulse rate, it is not too early to discuss your current level of fitness or lack of fitness.

If you feel you are more fit than you really are, you can very easily take on too much too soon, which can be discouraging.

On the other hand, if you feel you are terribly unfit, there could be a tendency to undermine your own efforts by being too cautious to accept new challenges.

In any fitness program, however, it is always best to err on the conservative side. It is better to do too little than too much.

Remember, also, that when dealing with fitness for those over 50, age is a very important factor. Your body has different limitations now than when you were 20.

I've broken the subjective evaluation down into five categories. Don't put pressure on yourself to shoe-horn yourself into a category where you think you should be. This is not a test. This is merely to start you thinking about your current perception of yourself. Read the five categories and put a check mark next to the one you feel best describes you now.

Level 1. Seldom walk at all. I tend to avoid walking or other forms of exercise. When it comes to doing errands, I always take the car or get a ride, even if it is merely a matter of a few blocks. I don't stroll or walk for pleasure. I feel that the term "sedentary" accurately describes me.

Level 2. Stroll and walk modestly. At least several times a week I take a stroll or a walk either alone or with one or more friends. I never walk fast, but I do walk, and I derive some enjoyment from it. My strolling and/or walking constitutes the extent of my exercise during the typical week. I never do either at a pace that would cause me to perspire or pant.

Level 3. Walk regularly. When I have to go on an errand within a reasonable distance, I tend to walk at an unhurried pace. I do this three to five times a week, and I enjoy occasionally taking a bit of a constitution after eating. I don't exert myself when I walk because I've been walking regularly long enough that there is little effort involved. I do consider it my exercise, however, and I also find it a good psychological outlet.

Level 4. I make it a habit to walk at least once a

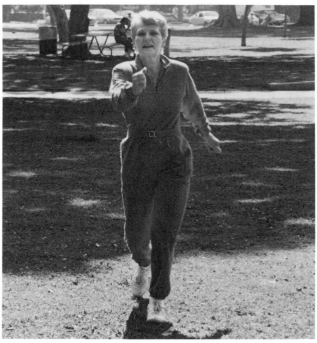

Going It Alone—Although it is fun to walk with others, if you have been diligently training to Dynastride better and faster, other people may tend to slow you down. I enjoy getting in a good Dynastriding workout with Jack, but I also enjoy going out on my own, where I can be alone with my own thoughts. You'd be surprised at all the seemingly stubborn problems that solve themselves when you take them out for a walk.

day, usually one or two miles at a time. I do my errands by walking, and although I have a car, if the weather is favorable and the distance I must go is not too far, I prefer walking over riding. I've been doing this for years and find it both invigorating and relaxing.

Level 5. I regularly walk vigorously. I see my walking as my primary exercise, and when I do it, I do it with vigor and determination. I walk as quickly as I can and as smoothly, while always staying within a safe pulse range; I stop every half-mile or so to take my pulse rate. I do this type of walking four to six times a week, and can go four to five miles at a time, although three to four is my usual daily walk. Occasionally I'll walk with friends at a more sedate pace.

Make certain you've made your check mark next to the level that best describes you. If, as you read this book, you find what I'm talking about makes sense, you'll be moving up the scale before you finish this book.

In the following chapters we'll describe what you need for a safe and successful walking program.

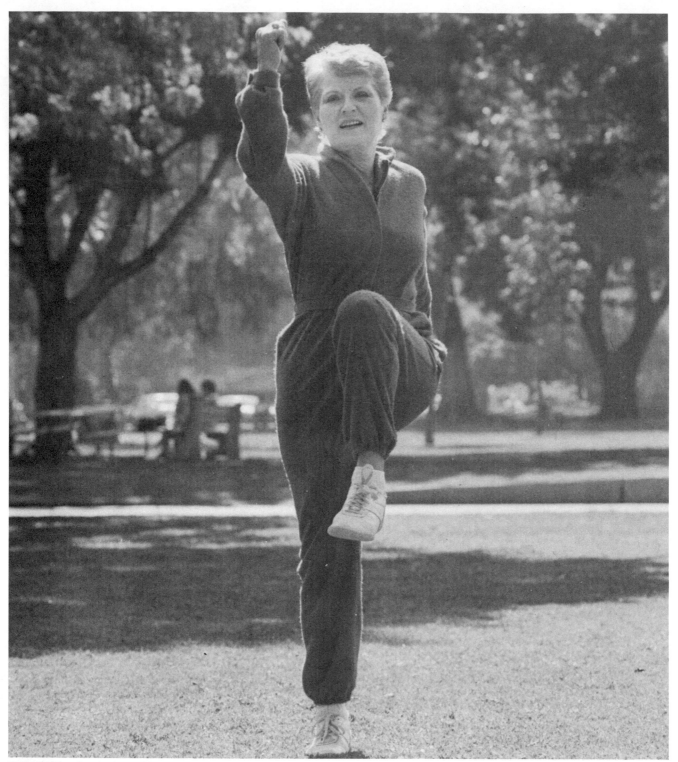

Mix It Up Occasionally—I use a high-stepping marching routine to begin my cool-down exercises, but I find that it also comes in handy as a way to further loosen up the big leg muscles during the middle of a walk. Try it sometime. Halfway through your Dynastride workout, go into a vigorous marching routine for about 10-12 steps, and then fall back into your Dynastriding. Notice how much more limber the big muscles in the legs feel during the second half of the workout.

Chapter 3

What's Needed For Safe And Sane Walking

"The sum of the whole is this: walk and be happy, walk and be healthy."
—Charles Dickens

It is important before embarking on an exercise program, especially if you are over 35 like most of us, to have a complete physical check-up, including a stress test. Why? Simple! To evaluate your current level of health and to spot irregularities of which you may not be aware: anything from high blood pressure to diabetes, elevated cholesterol to problems of coordination (that may point to a cerebral problem). When beginning a fitness program, the complete physical will provide you with a set of guidelines and may point out any weak areas which you must work around. That's the role of the check-up, even if you aren't taking up a fitness lifestyle.

Hopefully your doctor believes in and is knowledgeable of the numerous studies published in medical journals over the past decade lauding the various benefits of a regular program of physical activity. If he does not believe exercise is important, smokes, is excessively overweight or suffers any of the maladies of abuse that he warns you against, you might consider getting a second opinion (just as you would for your car, if you were not satisfied with the first estimate).

When you have completed your physical, your doctor will be able to give you a reasonable evalua-

tion of your current condition and will be able to point out things you should be aware of and cautions you should take in starting a walking program. Or, if you have kept yourself in relatively good health, your doctor may give you all green lights across the board and encourage you to get in there and start stepping lively.

For people over 50 who have not kept fit over the years, I have another recommendation. Schedule an examination by either a sports-oriented health-care professional or a podiatrist in order to evaluate the biomechanical efficiency of your legs, feet and back. You'll want to know if you have any existing problems and what you can do to minimize them. Should you have any problems, he will recommend or outline alternatives.

These problems, by the way, can be anything from chronic back or knee problems to stiffness in the legs, corns and bunions to hammertoes. Because of the huge number of people who began running in the 1970s, a great deal of research was done on the lower body, and a whole arsenal of solutions to foot and leg problems have come about as a result—everything from shoe inserts to stretching exercises.

As a child, I really never paid much attention to

my feet. But as I grew older, I noticed that they were getting harder and harder to fit. The salesperson would measure my right foot and suggest accordingly; however, my left foot always felt "squished" in the shoe, until I discovered it was a half size larger than my right. I then bought shoes a half size larger. However, my feet still felt cramped (especially around my bunions).

Believe it or not, it wasn't until I was in my 50s that I found out the "B" width (which most stores carry) was not for me or my feet. Hallelujah! I finally found a store that catered to people with wider feet (C width and larger). It was heaven! All these years suffering from sore feet, when something so simple as a wider shoe could have solved my problem.

One day when my feet and I were really in pain, I kicked off my shoes and set them side by side and noticed a "listing." In other words, the heels were worn on the outsides. I said to myself: "I'm walking on the outside of my feet—no wonder I have problems."

With all these revelations regarding my feet, I decided to get a medical opinion. I made an appointment with a wonderful podiatrist. I had visions of having foot surgery to correct the condition. My doctor evaluated the situation and suggested that we try an insert before we decided on anything more radical. He took casts of my feet and made orthotics for me, which I have been wearing ever since in my running, walking and golfing shoes.

Incredibly, some foot and leg problems that people over 50 experience are not due to using the feet and legs too much, but come from *not using them enough*. Remember that as you age, the calcium and other minerals in your bones can decrease and cause myriad problems. Several studies conducted over the past few years indicate that bone loss is due to lack of use. The studies also indicate that people who take up a regular exercise program help reverse the process, and instead of losing minerals, the bones begin to add calcium and other essential minerals, thereby making them stronger. Exercise benefits not only the bones of the feet and the legs, but all the bones in the body.

Another medical aspect of walking that I find fascinating is the incredible relief to the feet that many people who take up walking get simply from getting their feet into a good pair of walking shoes. It was common to see this happen when running shoes became popular. Older people who had had foot problems all their lives (often caused by chronically wearing shoes that were too tight or that offered no support) slipped on a pair of running shoes and felt like their feet had gone to heaven. It became almost impossible to get those people out of the running shoes. The same is even more true of walking shoes, due to the fact that the soles of well-designed walking shoes are rounded to set up an economical, comfortable rolling motion to the foot, making the entire process more pleasant. The newer walking shoes are also quite attractive and not as gaudy as some of the running shoes.

To reiterate:

1. Have a complete physical (including a stress test) and consult on the results of that physical with a sports-oriented health care professional who is knowledgeable concerning the benefits of modest exercise.

2. If you have even the slightest suspicion that you have any foot, leg or back abnormalities (and these *do* include bunions and corns and hammertoes), it would be worth your while before you start your walking program to meet with a sports-oriented health professional to learn how you can minimize problems from the parts of your body that will be doing most of the work.

Time and Where to Find It

When it comes to time, there are two kinds of people: those who feel there are too many hours in a day, and those who feel there aren't enough.

A regular walking program has benefits for both kinds of time-conscious people:

1. For those who feel the day drags too slowly, the half hour to one hour per day dedicated to your walking program not only will give you added energy and vitality but it will fill that time with something more productive. It will make the hours go by quickly and pleasantly and the process of walking may ultimately open new vistas that will tend to make each hour more precious.

2. If you are one of those people like myself who feels pressured to stuff as much into a day as possible, putting 30 minutes to an hour aside each day for walking can be like stopping off at a filling station. Why? Because the time spent exercising provides added energy stores in the body that will last for hours. If the time you spend walking is done over the lunch hour, you will probably find that you have more energy in the afternoon, the time of day our energy seems to be the lowest. Because of that phenomenon of additional energy from exercise, the hours in the day for the busy person will tend to be even more productive, more effective and energetically used, both mentally and physically.

When considering *when* to walk, remember that not all people are created alike. Because a friend of yours exercises first thing in the morning does not mean that the morning is the right time for you. Due to a complex system of circadian rhythms (natural rhythms of waking and sleeping), some people are best suited to do their exercise in the morning, while others do best in the early evening.

I like to compare people to some of our feathered friends: roosters and chickens (early morning people), skylarks (those who perform best in the middle of the day when the sun is high) and nightowls (who hit their stride after dark). You probably know which one you are, so try to arrange your walking to accommodate your body. The object, after all, is to make this exercise program an integral part of your life, not a punishment.

Keep these rules of foot in mind:

1. It is best to try to get in the habit of exercising at the same time each day so that walking becomes part of your regular routine. However, if it is impossible to be consistent, make sure you fit it in somewhere. As Jack says, "Something is better than nothing."

2. Aim to do some walking five to seven times a week. Again, this is because exercise works best when you are consistent.

3. Plan to fit your walking into times and circumstances where it complements other things you are doing that day. Do you have to drop your car off to have the engine tuned? Why not drop it off, take the bus home, and when it's time to go pick the car up, use that as your walk? Or, can you use your walking to get to your luncheon appointment or to visit a friend? Remember that the wonderful thing about walking is that, barring extremely hot weather, you can walk briskly and get your exercising in without having to change into special exercise clothes before you walk, change out of your special exercise clothes after you walk, and then take a shower before getting back into your regular clothes. Much of the walking you do will be brisk but far from exhausting, and will require no special clothing, making it the most convenient of all exercises to fit into your day.

These Shoes Were Made for Walking

One of the beauties of running has always been its simplicity. In order to run, a person did not have to purchase a lot of equipment or find a partner or a team. The runner merely bought a pair of good running shoes, changed into a pair of shorts and a T-shirt, and was out the door; upon the return, the runner would shower and change back into civilian clothes.

Hard as it is to believe, walking is even easier. And even less expensive.

For the most part, the walker doesn't even have to buy a pair of shorts; most walking can be done in comfortable clothing that you already own. And there is usually no need to shower and change again after you're finished with your walking, unless it was a particularly long walk or unless the walk was done on a particularly hot day.

The only investment of any significance that faces the walker is a pair of good walking shoes. And at the start, most people can even put that off for a few weeks—although it isn't advised.

Walking, if it is to be taken up with dedication and turned into a regular part of your day, demands its own shoes.

You may feel that you already have a comfortable pair of shoes in which you walk. Or you may have purchased a pair of the very comfortable running shoes that make your tired feet feel so good.

Shoes that are comfortable for walking around the house and down the street may not be constructed to give your feet support over the long haul. Casual shoes may be all right for casual strolling about, but are usually not adequate for real walking.

The problem with running shoes is that they are designed for *running*, with a good deal of support built into the heels, where most long-distance runners first impact with the ground. These shoes are built for striking the ground and then toeing off: for impact and rebound.

A good pair of walking shoes is constructed to absorb your impact with the ground, yes, but not to the extent that a running shoe is. Instead of being built to rebound you after your impact, a good walking shoe is built to facilitate your *rolling* forward into your toe-off.

Many people who have found running shoes wonderfully comfortable after a lifetime of squeezing and forcing their feet into hard shoes or shoes that were in fashion but that offered no real comfort may want to begin their walking program by sticking with their running shoes. If the shoes are comfortable and have given you no problems,

that's fine. It isn't perfect, but if your feet are comfortable, that's the important thing.

If you don't have a pair of running shoes in the closet, however, it would be best to get broken in immediately on the shoe designed specifically for walking.

There are a few areas of shoe construction you'll want to keep in mind when shopping for a pair of walking shoes:

1. Be certain that there are no knots or rough edges *inside* the shoe that will cause blisters or that will bother you when you walk. A well-made pair of walking shoes will feel smooth inside. You may be able to discern seams when you put your hand inside, but the seams should be recessed and free of protrusions that could irritate your foot.

2. A good shoe will have a stiff heel counter. This is the portion of the shoe that wraps around your heel. To determine a properly stiff heel counter, hold the shoe in one hand, and with your free hand, grasp the two sides of the back of the shoe that support the heel. Squeeze the two sides to-

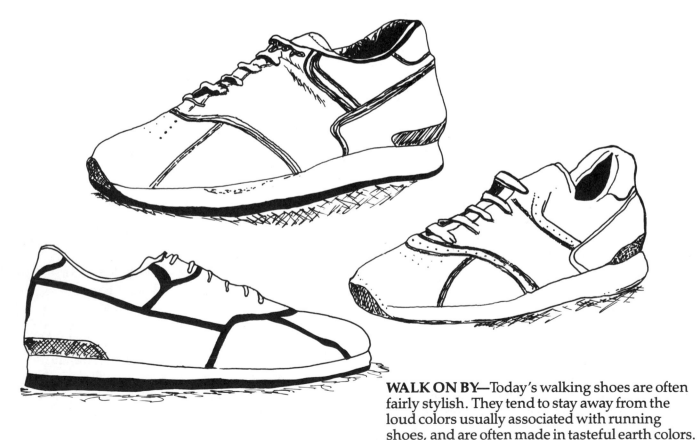

WALK ON BY—Today's walking shoes are often fairly stylish. They tend to stay away from the loud colors usually associated with running shoes, and are often made in tasteful earth colors.

gether. A good heel counter should offer significant resistance.

3. The next important consideration is the toe box, the front that will house your toes. Make certain that you can wiggle your toes around freely. You do not want to feel the sides of the shoe impinging on the sides of your big or little toe, and you want about an inch of free space in front of your toes. This inch of empty space is needed for several reasons:

• When you walk for any length of time, your feet begin to expand because of increased blood supply to the working muscles and because of minor swelling.

• When you are walking down a hill, there will be a tendency for your foot to slide forward a bit. You don't want the toes, under those circumstances, to make contact with the front of the shoe, or the contact will irritate your toes and could cause discomfort.

4. A good shoe is as wide as your foot. Many modern shoe manufacturers make their walking shoes in varying widths. Don't force your wide foot into a narrow shoe. And don't allow your narrow foot to slide around in a wide shoe. Never make your foot fit a shoe's dimensions.

5. Never, but *never* buy a pair of slip-on or loafer type walking shoes. Always buy lace shoes. This allows for a better fit, better support, less sliding of the foot inside the shoe, and allows you to make adjustments to the fit of the shoe by tightening or loosening the laces. Also, slip-on type shoes put your toes through a great deal of extra work. Your toes must be gripping the front inside of the shoe to prevent the shoe from slipping. This can, over the long haul, cause blisters and a variety of other problems.

With the revolution in walking (just as in the revolution in running before it), the marketplace has responded. Many of the companies that helped bring the running shoe into the 20th century are now designing good walking shoes.

When I meet people on my walks, one of their first questions to me concerns shoes. "What walking shoe is best for me?" they'll ask. What I've found is that since every foot is different, each foot adapts differently to a specific shoe. Try out a variety of brands and models until you find one that fits well and provides good support and cushioning.

You can expect to pay between $30 and $100 a pair for walking shoes, but a good pair will serve you well and will last a considerably longer time than a cheap knock-off that may cause foot problems.

If you currently have foot problems, it would be best to schedule an appointment with your podiatrist before you go shopping. Your foot doctor may suggest an insert or orthotic to take care of a foot problem, such as I have. You'll need to find a shoe that will accommodate the insert. Sometimes this involves buying a shoe a half-size larger than normal in order to have room to accommodate it. If you use an orthotic, take that along with you when you try on shoes.

Remember, too, it is always best to go shopping for shoes late in the day, when your feet have already had all day long to swell as much as they are going to.

And since you are going to wear socks when you do your walking exercises, use the same socks you will wear to walk when you try on your new shoes. Your socks should be absorbent but not bulky. And don't wear tube socks or the one-size-fits-all. Wear socks that are just a mite longer than your foot. Cotton socks are good and wool socks are usually acceptable, especially if you live in a cold climate. Some of the blends of cotton and synthetic fibers are also good.

When you go to shop for shoes, don't buy the first pair you try on. Try on a variety of shoes; walk around in them in the store. If this is the first time you've shopped for walking shoes, the tendency is going to be to want to buy the first pair you try on because they generally feel so much more comfortable than your everyday shoes. Be patient. Remember, though, that these shoes must carry you hundreds of miles, so take your time to get your proper fit. If you are uncertain after walking around in the store with the shoes on, pick the pair you feel most comfortable in, pay for them but be sure that you can return them if they don't feel the same at home. When you get them home, wear them around the house for an hour or so. Don't

WALKING SHOE

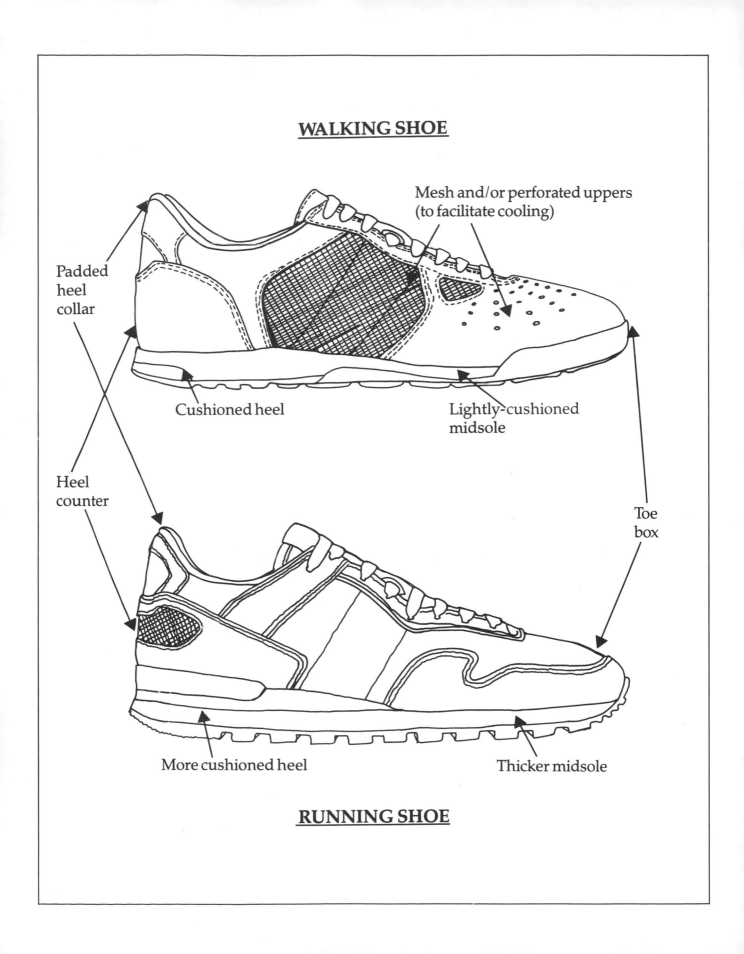

Mesh and/or perforated uppers
(to facilitate cooling)

Padded
heel
collar

Cushioned heel

Lightly-cushioned
midsole

Heel
counter

Toe
box

More cushioned heel

Thicker midsole

RUNNING SHOE

wear them outside, however. You don't want to scuff them up. It would be unfair to attempt to return a pair of shoes you'd scuffed to the point they can't be resold to someone else.

Most walking shoes are made of leather. But some (of lighter weight) have fabric uppers.

Leather usually wears longer but is heavier and must generally be broken in a bit. Do not buy shoes made of patent leather, however, because such shoes do not breathe well.

Fabric uppers have the benefit of being light-weight and they dry quickly and breathe well. They are not very good for cold climates, however, because they allow cold air to come through the uppers. And they generally do not hold up as long as leather uppers.

Some companies are making walking shoes that are primarily leather but that feature fabric panels at flex points.

It is generally best to go with what feels best to you. But *do* keep in mind that if you do walk in cold weather that features slushy streets, leather is generally best, although it *will* take longer to dry afterwards than fabric.

It might be worth your while to look for a specialty store that deals with runners and features a line or two of walking shoes; or check into an outdoors shop if your area has one: a shop that sells hiking boots and tents and sleeping bags and that caters to backpackers instead of hunters. If they carry a line or two of walking shoes, you're more likely to find a salesperson who knows something about walking.

If you don't get a satisfactory response, move on until you find someone who does some serious walking themselves.

Once you have your shoes, you'll want to keep them in good condition. This involves *always* wearing socks when you use your shoes. And keep your socks clean. Salts in your sweat and acids from your feet can wear out a good pair of shoes very fast; by wearing socks, the perspiration is trapped and the life of the shoes extended significantly.

Also, if your shoes get wet, don't dry them by putting them too close to a source of heat. This applies to both leather and fabric shoes. If your shoes are wet, take them off and stuff them with bunched up newspaper and then set them at a warm, dry spot to dry.

This brings up another important point. If you can possibly afford it, two pair of walking shoes are about 10 times better than one. If one pair gets wet, you can wear the alternate pair while the wet pair dries. Plus, alternating shoes further extends the life of the shoes. It also extends the life of your feet. Walking in the same pair of shoes every day can aggravate foot problems because muscles and joints are taking impacts at the same exact angle, day after day. By alternating shoes, the impact can be spread over more area of the bones and tendons and muscles; this avoids consistently stressing your legs, ankles and feet over and over in the same, exact way.

The science of shoes has advanced so tremendously over the past decade that there's been no better time in history to go shopping for a good pair.

Clothes for Comfortable Walking

If you already own clothing that is loose-fitting and comfortable, there is probably no need to even contemplate purchasing additional clothing for walking. Loose-fitting clothing does not restrict movement, while tight-fitting clothing can make virtually any type of exercise more difficult and uncomfortable.

For mild weather, a pair of slacks and a comfortable T-shirt or open-neck shirt or blouse is usually all that's needed. If the weather is changeable, it is best to take along a water-repellant jacket or an umbrella, of course. Since most of the walks in my program are of less than an hour's duration, don't be caught by surprise by errant weather patterns.

I also recommend wearing a hat, no matter what the weather. In warm weather, the hat should be light-colored and should be mesh or in some other way breathable; you don't want to have the sun beating down on a bare head. In cold weather, a hat of warm construction is best. Approximately half of the heat the body loses escapes through the head. The object is to allow it to escape on warm weather walks and to retain much of it on cold weather walks.

In warm weather, it is best to wear light-colored clothing, white if possible, because it will reflect away the sunshine and keep you cooler. You should also wear clothing that is fairly breathable in order to allow the circulation of air to dry perspiration and cool the body.

In cold weather, dress in layers instead of one very thick piece of clothing. (There are several reasons for this.) Once you begin your walk, your body will begin producing heat, so you will be warmer in the middle of your walk than at the beginning, and it will be difficult to adjust your body temperature if you are wearing only one bulky garment. If you are dressed in layers, you can remove one layer in order to become more comfortable, or easily put that layer back on. As you remove a layer of clothing, tie the jacket around your waist instead of restricting the movement of your arms while walking. The other reason to dress in layers is that the body warmth is trapped in the air spaces between layers, serving as insulation to keep you warm.

Once you've really gotten into walking, you may want to invest in a warm-up suit or in one of the more weatherproof Gore-Tex outfits. Many of these exercise garments are made in very contemporary designs, and they are quite comfortable, especially for walking. Although expensive, Gore-Tex is a special material that allows your body heat and perspiration to escape through the material, while preventing the droplets of rain from penetrating.

When buying a workout outfit for walking, I always advise looking for one that is either very bright or that comes with reflective panels sewn into it. After all, you're most likely to want to use such an outfit when the weather is foul, which is also when visibility is at its worst. Give motorists every chance in the world to see you as you walk your way to health.

Nutrition Is Important, Too

"God gave the Americans the greatest food in the world and the devil came along and invented the frying pan." That's another Jack LaLannism that fits well here.

An entire book could be written about the importance of nutrition for the over-50 exerciser and athlete. But I'm going to keep this section brief, since there are some general rules that, if followed, will help your program—and your health in general—greatly.

Remember this: a regular exercise program combined with good nutrition causes fat loss. As a nation, we are overfed and undernourished; we eat way too much fat and not enough fiber. Saturated fats, as most of us know, are butter, shortenings, some margarines and oils (read the labels), dairy products such as whole milk, cheese, and sour cream. Also much of our baked goods made with shortening are high in saturated fats. A diet high in saturated fats can lead to not only increased weight but increased cholesterol, high blood pressure, hardening of the arteries, diabetes, heart disease, stroke and even some forms of cancer.

What can we do about this? We can cut down on our fat intake and burn it up through exercise. Many people like to take the easy way out and look for a magic pill or potion that will make them lose weight. Remember that exercise and nutrition go hand-in-hand. If you are taking in more calories than you are burning up, that weight isn't going to come off as readily.

Suppose you had a piece of paper and you wanted it to disappear. How would you do it? You could crumple it, stomp on it, roll it up in a ball, but it would still be there. The only way to get rid of it would be to burn it. The same with fat in our body. Exercise helps burn fat. Long endurance activities, such as Dynastriding or slow jogging helps burn fat best. What better way to start burning fat than to walk?

"But," you say, "we need fat in our bodies." Yes, we do, but most of us get twice as much as we need. When we exercise we burn fat, which produces energy. However, it is more difficult to turn calories stored in the body from saturated fats into ready energy than it is for those from complex carbohydrates. So, for ready energy, start using more complex carbohydrates such as fresh fruits, fresh vegetables and whole grains. The fiber from these will also fill you up faster—fill you up and not out.

Cut back on high fat foods, trim fats from meat and avoid marbled cuts; if you are making chicken, remove the skin, and try to eat more fish. Learn to read labels. (Many packaged foods have high fat content.) Learn to enjoy food you have never eaten before. Variety is the key to good natural eating. Learn to chew your food; the slower you chew your food, the less you are going to want to eat. Always eat when you are relaxed; avoid eating when you are upset. Try to refrain from eating white flour and white sugar products and eat foods in their natural states as much as possible; don't overindulge. Moderation should be your motto.

If I've heard Jack say this once, I've heard him say it a hundred times: "It's not what you do some of the time, but what you do most of the time that counts."

Then there's water. Very few people I know drink enough water. The sedentary adult should drink two quarts of water a day. The adult who is exercising should drink more. Water assists in regularity and it is essential for cell repair; it is also essential for cooling the exercising body. Do not be afraid to take a glass of water before you start your walk and after you complete it. Even in cold weather, the exercising body loses water, so don't forget to replace it.

Your walking should be scheduled before meals, if at all possible. This has two good effects. It allows the blood to be diverted to the working muscles (in this case, the legs) and it tends to curb your appetite so that when you sit down to eat, you won't be quite as hungry. I don't recommend exercising vigorously directly after eating because your body's blood is being diverted to the stomach to help digest the food. It is all right to take a stroll after eating, but when we talk about walking in this book, we're referring to Dynastriding or vigorous walking for the whole body.

If you are on prescription drugs, check with your doctor to be certain that a regular exercising program is safe for you. In most instances, exercise will have no negative effects upon prescription drugs, but is worth a phone call to check.

Many people ask me what I think of coffee. It seems that for every study that comes out telling us how caffeine is bad for us, another one comes out telling us it can have good effects if taken in moderation. My advice would be that if you have been drinking coffee regularly and have had no ill effects, it probably won't hurt now just because you are exercising. If in doubt, check with your doctor. If you are not currently drinking coffee, I won't recommend starting now. I would suggest, however, to take more vitamin E because caffeine helps deplete the vitamin E in your system just like smoking depletes vitamin C and sugar and alcohol depletes vitamin B.

Extra Equipment: . . . What Will They Think of Next?

With every movement of any size that comes down the pike, it seems that a virtual army of marketeers comes forward to sell and profit from that movement.

Some of the products created for the emerging market are essential, some are potentially useful, and some totally useless.

As we've already discussed, the only equipment you literally need for walking is a good, comfortable, functional pair of shoes.

Beyond the shoes, a watch is useful, as long as it has a second hand. The watch is needed for reminding yourself on an out-and-back course when it is time to turn around to come back. The second hand is essential in monitoring your pulse rate.

Beyond the shoes and watch, the most useful pieces of equipment you might care to invest in (and it is a small investment at that) is either a laminated I.D. card (with appropriate medical information listed) and/or a Medical Alert necklace or bracelet where needed.

If you do your walking before sun-up or when it's dark, it would also be worth investing in a reflective vest so that automobile traffic can see you.

Pedometers are fun but sometimes can be inaccurate because one person's stride might be 18 inches while another is 24 inches. You see, the pedometer measures the distance you walk by the number of strides you take. Your stride may be 16 inches during the first half mile (while the muscles are still cold) and 24 inches by the end of your walk (when the legs warm up).

What about wrist, waist, vest and/or ankle weights? Although they do cause you to burn a few more calories, most people over 50 do not need the extra weight—at least at the beginning of a program. The weight can alter your natural stride and arm swing. Also, if you are a beginner, it can place extra stress on the legs, ankles and feet. I would suggest leaving them for the more proficient walker.

Walkman type radios are up to the individual but can be distracting and muffle the sound of approaching traffic.

Walking sticks can be useful for walking uphill or downhill, poking around in the grass, or walking in a territory of unleashed dogs. However, it certainly isn't a mandatory piece of equipment. If you don't want to invest in a walking stick you can whittle one yourself. Or, for protection, go to your local junkyard and pick up a telescoping antenna from a damaged car. I know of one man who walks with a baseball bat slung over his shoulder; a Louisville Slugger is good for leaning on, for discouraging pesky dogs, and for impressing the passing throng.

My yardstick for measuring the usefulness of a piece of equipment designed to enhance the walking experience is a simple question: "Will it improve my walking?"

Remember, the reason you've considered walking as your form of exercise is because of its simplicity. Keep it simple, and it will simply change your life for the better.

Chapter 4

Where And When?

"Take long walks in stormy weather or through deep snow in the fields and woods, if you would keep your spirits up."
—Henry David Thoreau

Whenever I hear my husband Jack speak—on an interview show, at a lecture, or just talking to friends—he inevitably brings up the fact that anything is possible in life if you put your mind to it. He strongly believes that we all need challenges in our lives. And just because we are older and maybe even retired does not mean that we should give up accepting new challenges and approaching them creatively! In my mind I can even now hear him ending one of his lectures with this message: "ANYTHING IS POSSIBLE IN LIFE. MAKE IT HAPPEN!"

As I sit here writing this chapter, I'd like to ask you a question: How is it possible to fit a regular walking program into your life? At the same time, I challenge you to do it.

You know as well as I do that if we have the desire to do something, such as go to the store and buy this book, we are never too busy to make use of that desire to get things accomplished.

Isn't it wonderful that each one of us is a unique individual in this great universe of ours, and each one of us looks at life quite differently? We each have different needs and wishes. We have varied schedules, and as a result, what works perfectly for Gertrude in Sarasota, Florida will not necessarily work for Jim in Seattle, Washington. The circumstances under which a walking program is successfully initiated might even be radically different for two people in a town of 200 in Missouri.

I *am* certain, however, that if I were to bounce this topic into your court, I'd be astounded by the creativity that you would exhibit. To get your mind working in the direction of how you can best fit walking into your daily life, here are a few examples:

—A friend of mine who works around the house most of the day came up with a unique solution. He measured off a circuit of the inside of his house, both upstairs and downstairs, making a circuit of each room, and by being very creative, he came up with a mile course. So, when the clock tells him it's time for his workout, he doesn't even have to leave the house. He merely follows the course through the house for the prescribed amount of time that day and then records the results in his journal. The fact that he uses both floors of his house is a bonus: he manages to add some hillwork (climbing the stairs) to every workout.

—Another friend who is very good at organizing time lives in a town with a very distinct downtown shopping area. Over breakfast every morning she plans all of her errands on a Xerox of the downtown area; she works out a route that will accomplish all of her errands while creating a walk that will keep her going for the prescribed amount of time that day. She is careful not to linger at any one location because the object is to keep your pulse rate up. Instead, she keeps it short and sweet, and uses the slight pauses along the way to take her pulse rate. She is so efficient at her errands that her pulse never drops out of her target area. She reports that this method of running errands is a wonderful cure for shopping because in order to get her workout in, she can't afford time to stop and look at anything the stores are trying to sell her.

—Quite a few of my friends and acquaintances combine their walk with walking their dog. That way, they accomplish two things at once. An added benefit, for both dog and owner, is that they both get more exercise than before, and both show the benefits in fat loss, muscle tone and that feeling-younger glow. I walk with our dog, Happy. No, he is not the same white Happy you saw on TV years ago. That Happy has gone to dog heaven. Zsa Zsa Gabor, who loves dogs, gave us a son of her black German shepherd several years ago and we named him Happy IV. He is all black and loves to play ball. Happy and I go walking every morning and he really keeps me going at a great pace. If he has his ball on our walk, I get in a lot of extra arm action, too.

Those are just a few creative methods of fitting the walking regime into one's day that I know of from friends who've taken up walking. I present them merely to jog your creativity. With a little imagination, it is often surprisingly easy to find a place for your walk within your normal day that causes a minimum of interference with your daily routine. Ultimately, that little walk you take will assume the aspect of a jewel in the crown of every day you live.

When planning how to fit your walk into your typical day, keep in mind that incidental walking around (walking out to the mailbox, for example) does not count toward your workout. In order to be of any real benefit, the walking must be sustained and continuous. Those short, little jaunts *do* add up, certainly, but never confuse them with a real workout. Think of them as additional adornment to your crown for that day. Trust me when I tell you that once you work a regular exercise walk into your day, you'll begin to automatically walk whenever the place you're going is within a reasonable distance. It will become like an automatic response. And in the instance of short-distance errands, you'll probably find that walking to and from your destination is often time-saving. Many people ultimately find that by just walking out the door to do errands, they can get there and back in much less time than it takes to start up the car, back it out of the driveway, drive it to the destination, find a parking place, turn it off, lock the car, and go inside.

Remember that when you are figuring out where in your day to place your walk, go with whatever time of day feels physically best for you and build upon that. You'll make walking easier on yourself, and you'll find that your good time of the day eventually begins to spread out over more and more hours, until it eventually infects your whole day with good feelings and accomplishments.

And don't be afraid to allow the creative side of you to come out in making those walking plans.

How to Create Your Courses

Don't undermine your fitness program by making it monotonous. A boring fitness program is guaranteed to cause you to give up. Unfortunately, this is what too often happens. Plus the fact that sometimes we try to do too much too soon. I'm sure this has happened to you or some of your friends.

It isn't the fitness that is monotonous, it is the approach of the people that can make it monotonous. Fitness is your servant. It will do what you tell it to do. Only *you* can make it boring. *But*, on the other hand, it is also *you* who can make it interesting.

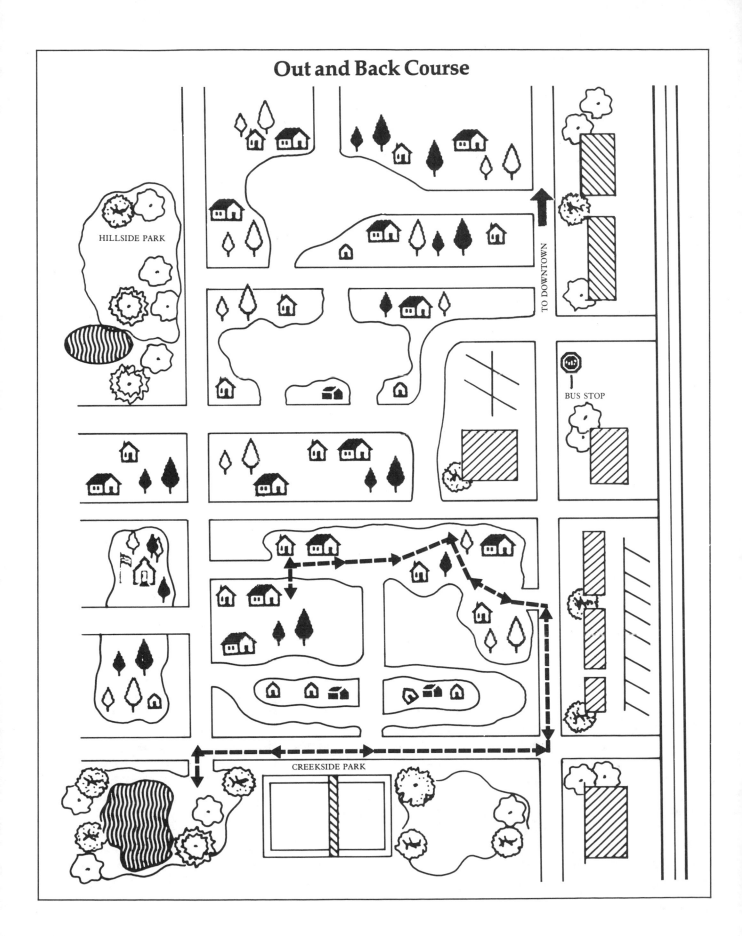

Out and Back Course

HILLSIDE PARK

TO DOWNTOWN

BUS STOP

CREEKSIDE PARK

And you don't have to make it extremely complex to make it interesting. Your goal, after all, is to make your walking program a comfortable part of your typical day. Your walk should ultimately be something you look forward to, not something you dread.

Even long-term fitness addicts can become bored with their workouts if there is no variety. Add variety and creativity, and even the most bored exerciser can be revived.

Don't wait to become burned out. Vary your routine from the very outset and boredom will never become an issue.

If variety is the spice of life, it is also the spice of my walking program. No two days in a row are alike. As a result, you will find it necessary to devise a variety of courses right from the start.

Let's discuss the kind of courses that you can create. They fall into various categories:

Out and Back This is the most basic and simple of all courses, and is one that is most often used to begin your program. It is also of great use if you are traveling and you end up in strange territory and want to get your workout accomplished that day. It is merely a walk away from your house or your motel room in a direction that looks interesting, with a time goal in mind; when you reach half of your time goal, you turn around and walk back. Simple, right? The only additional piece of information that is needed with this type of course is that if it is windy, start by walking into the wind so that the wind is at your back when you turn around to come back; there is no sense struggling into a headwind when you are tired during the second half of your walk.

Loop This couldn't be easier. You start and finish at the same spot by walking in a loop. This doesn't necessarily have to be a round loop. It can also be square. For instance, a circuit of the block in which your house is located is a loop course. As you become stronger and your walks increase in size, you may walk around two or three or 10 blocks. If you circle those blocks, it constitutes a loop course. A loop course is any course that essentially takes you around the edge of something (no matter what the shape) and deposits you back where you started.

Figure-8 The typical figure-8 is a course that joins two loops. Your house may be located at the juncture of the two loops or it could be at one of the ends. This course is noted by the fact that at some point in the walk, you cross (usually perpendicularly) a spot you've already walked. The two loops of a figure-8 do not have to be of equal size, by the way.

Point to Point This is a course where you start at one spot and finish at another. It does not have to be a course in a straight line, but it does obviously require that you employ some sort of transportation such as a car, bus or street car in one direction. It can be a walk home from downtown, where you had a medical appointment and took the bus. Or perhaps you walked from home to the park and did one loop of the park and then took a bus home. This type course is usually employed farther along in the program when you want to work your walking into your daily chores or errands or when you want to have an adventure with your walking.

Random Course A random course is merely one where you are walking for time and where you wander wherever your inclination takes you. To successfully do a random course, of course, you must know the neighborhood, because you want to end up back home by the end of your allotted time. I wouldn't suggest trying a random course in an unfamiliar environment. It becomes too easy to become disoriented and lost.

Geometric Course As you improve and can walk farther and farther, the geometric course can be one of the most interesting and fun variations because it is a course that you can continually add to: the pattern of the course becomes more complex and interesting the farther you go.

The beauty of all these types of courses is that you can create them so that every walk begins and ends at or near your front door (even the point-to-point if there's a bus stop nearby). My advice would be to get a map of your town and paste it on the bulletin board or on the refrigerator door, and plot courses on the street map in different colors. See how many different courses you can come up

Loop Course

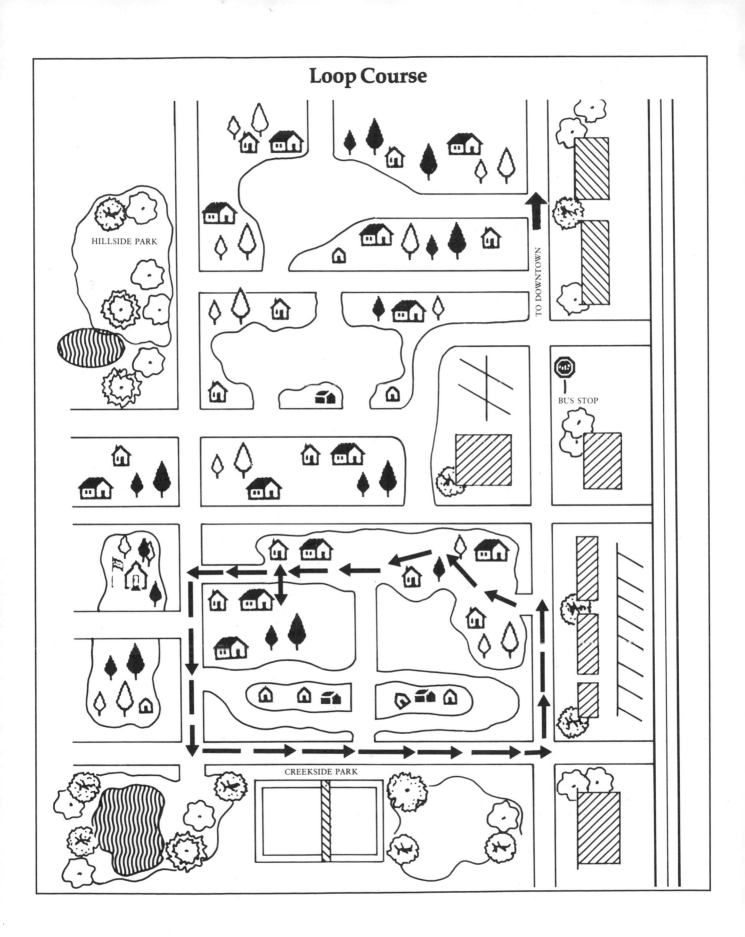

Figure-8 Course

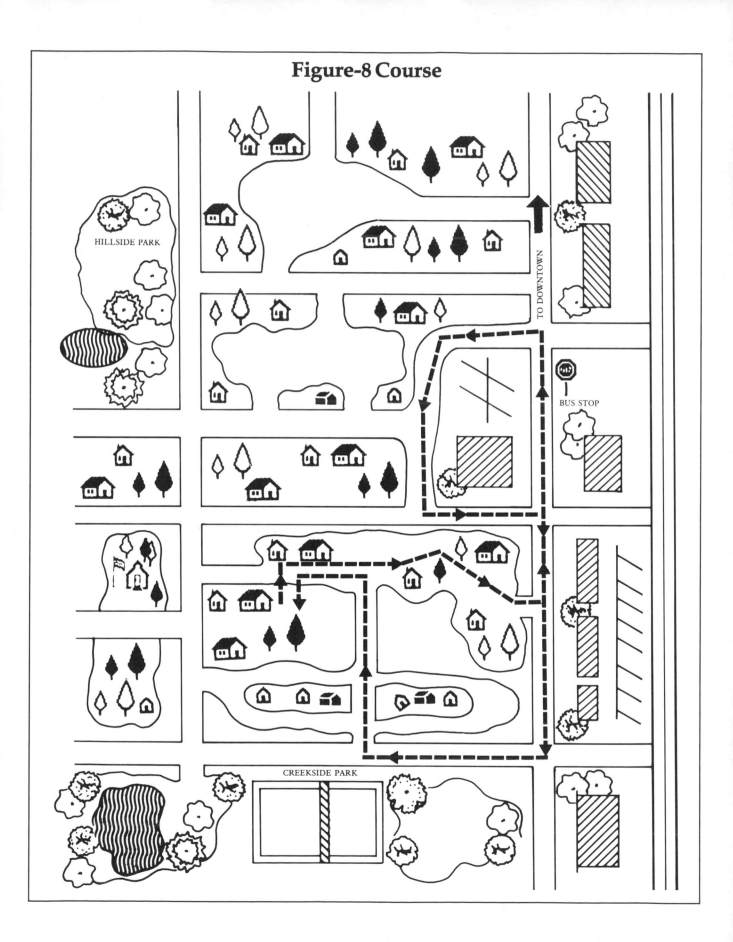

Point to Point Course

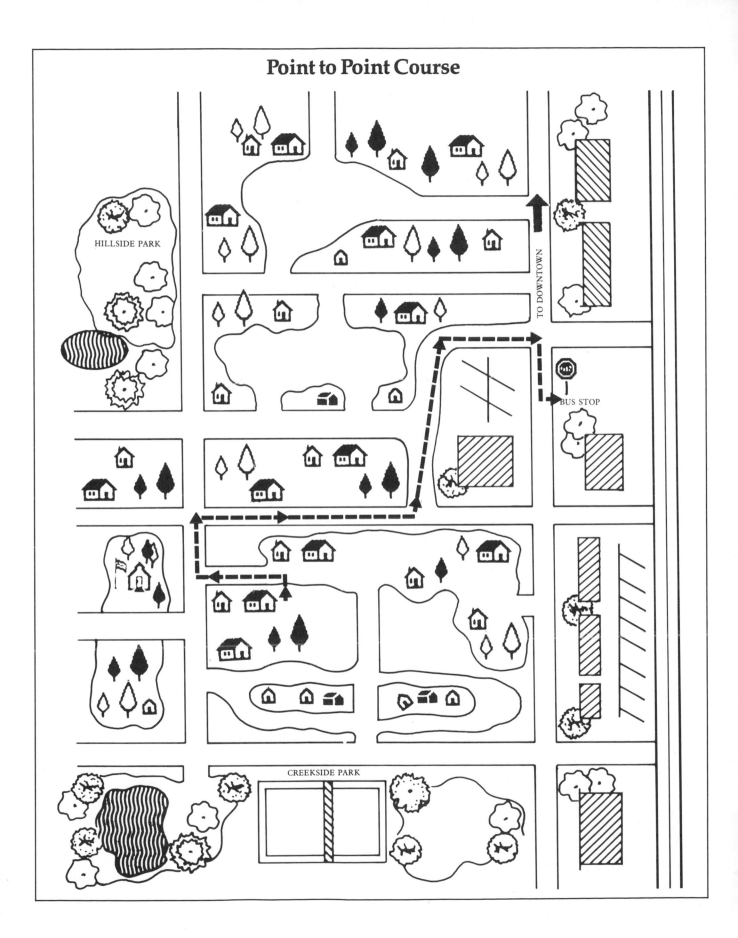

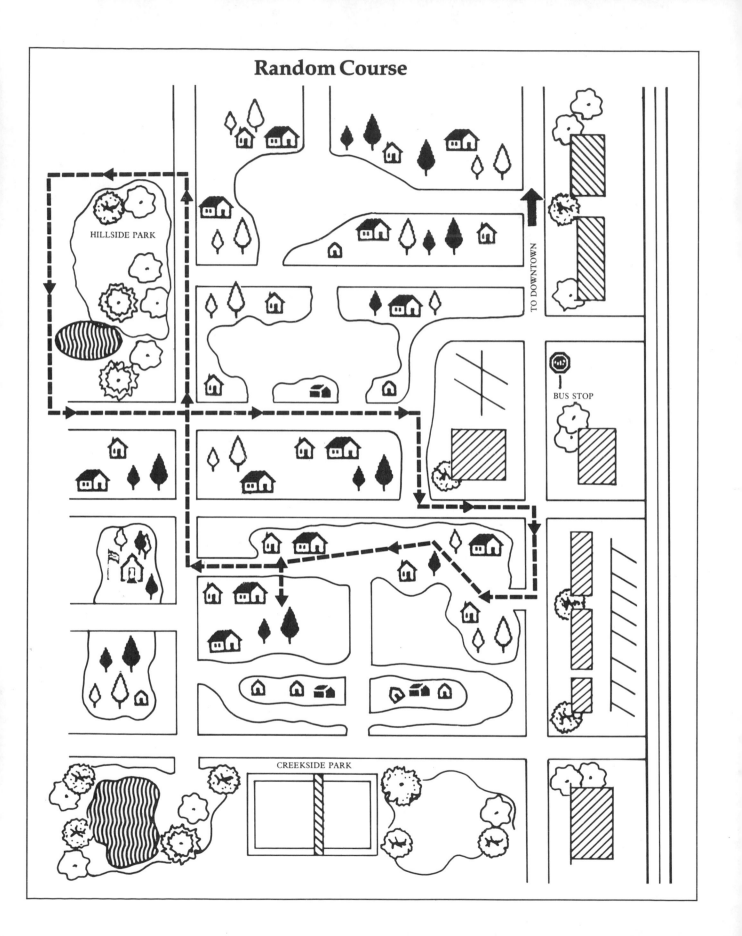

Random Course

HILLSIDE PARK

TO DOWNTOWN

BUS STOP

CREEKSIDE PARK

Geometric Course

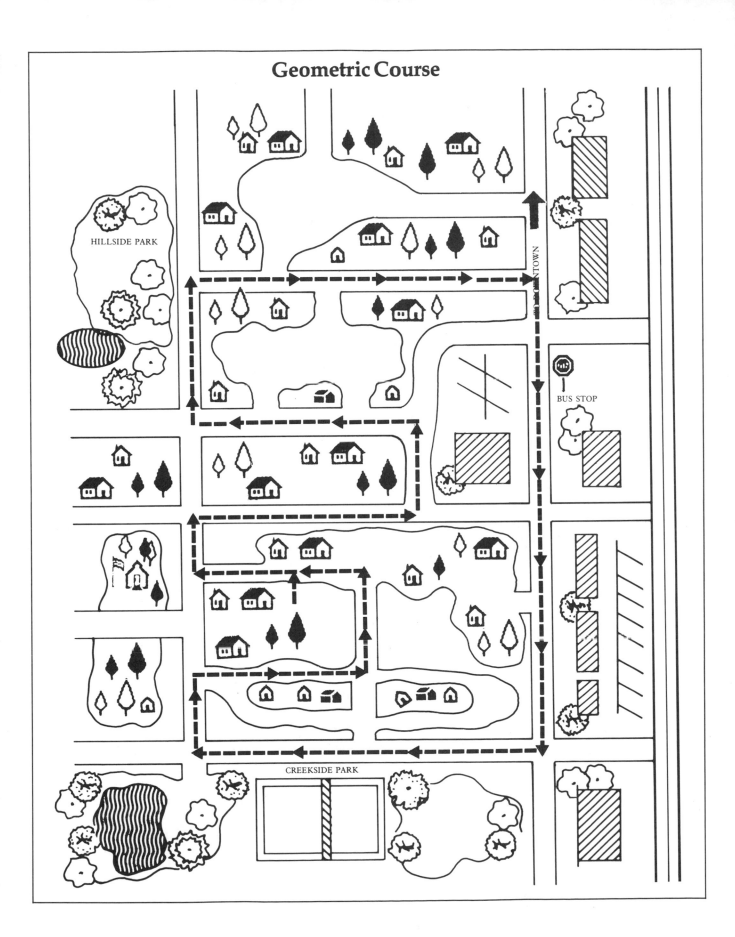

with merely by creating one each of the six different types of courses we've just discussed. Remember that each of those courses will grow as you become more fit and more able to go longer.

This method of adding on one more block at a time to a course as you become more able to go longer works well in a city or in the suburbs. It is not quite as easy when you live in the country because the countryside may have only one or two basic roads going by. The country dweller, however, can usually find little side roads or agreeable neighbors who don't mind if you wander on their land during your walks.

In either instance, however, as you become more able to walk well, you can also become creative by stringing together various courses in order to make super-courses or mega-courses.

When you walk in cities or suburbs, remember to walk on sidewalks whenever available. Don't walk along the roadway if you can help it. Besides, on heavily traveled roadways, the automobile exhaust lingers in the air, and who wants to breathe such bad air? If you find you must walk along roadways that are heavily traveled, walk toward traffic so that you can see the oncoming automobiles and so that they can see you. And wear bright, very easily-distinguished clothing. If you must walk along a roadway, the best times are early in the morning (before automobile exhaust pollution begins to thicken) or in the evening (when pollution has begun to thin out following the rush hour and when the cooling air disperses it). Never walk along a heavily-traveled roadway during the height of a sunny day; the sun causes additional chemical changes in the exhaust fumes, making them even more potent.

And don't become concerned with accurately measuring your courses, since my entire program is based upon time and pulse rate and not upon distance.

You can also create variety in your courses by inviting your friends to occasionally walk with you. Or, if you have several friends who also walk, visit them and walk on their courses occasionally. (You'll have to make certain to have walking friends who are similar to you in abilities, however, so that you can both get the benefits from the walk in terms of time and increased pulse rates.)

The Perfect Environment: Mall Walking

In areas of the country that experience foul weather (snow and sleet in the winter and dangerous heat combined with humidity in the summer), why not take up mall walking? If the weather is just dreadful outside, go to the local mall and walk inside the mall. Most malls are carefully temperature controlled and they are a safe environment: no automobiles to either choke you with pollution or run you down. And most of them are served by city bus lines.

Many malls accommodate walkers by opening several hours early so that people interested in walking can use the mall before the stores open and the crowds appear. Others have gone so far as to mark off distances inside the mall, or even sponsor regular walking groups.

There are some malls that have satellite health facilities inside where you can go to get your blood pressure taken and where you can join up with regular walking groups.

One such facility is A Measure of Wellness at The Courtyard Mall in Rolling Hills Estates near San Pedro in southern California, where I did my first mall walk lecture. A Measure of Wellness is a community health resource center (located on the mall's third floor) sponsored by San Pedro Peninsula Hospital. The walking course through the mall is marked every 1/6th of a mile, and A Measure of Wellness offices are open so that walkers can come in for a free blood pressure check. The center also features a wealth of information on everything from the dangers of smoking to obesity. It provides health and fitness screening (including a self-test which is done by computer), pamphlets and brochures on all aspects of health and fitness, films, books for loan, and a free call-in service called Tel Med where you can receive a pre-recorded message on literally hundreds of health topics: anemia, arthritis, cancer of the skin, diet tips for dental health, laxatives, etc. A Measure of Wellness also sponsors group walking activities at the mall and at nearby park locations for those who feel more comfortable doing their walking with a group.

Check with some of the hospitals in your area to see if they offer similar programs.

As interest in walking grows, more and more of the country's malls will see the wisdom in offering such programs and facilities. After all, the business of the mall owners is to get customers to come by. And a group of walkers doing a mile or two inside the mall constitutes quite a bit of window shopping for the merchants.

Let's move back to your creativity for a moment more. Why not begin to think of courses you could create both for yourself and for your friends when you get together for group walks? Here are a few suggestions:

—A walk that takes in some of the town's best-kept and most beautiful gardens.

—A course that connects all the gasoline stations or new car dealerships or pet shops or supermarkets, etc. in the vicinity.

—A course that creates a unique pattern when it is overlayed on a street map of the town.

—A course that connects various historic sites in town.

—If your town is built on a river, it is often nice to do an out-and-back walk along the river's edge, or to walk both sides of the river if there is a bridge available. As you become stronger, you'll reach a point farther up or down the river each time. A nice river walk every week or two is a very refreshing change. Keep your eyes open for wildlife along the way.

—As you become stronger and heartier, you can take free-form walks. Just head off, an apple in your pocket, and walk aimlessly, allowing your feet to guide you. (Again, the only caution here is to do this type of walking in neighborhoods with which you are familiar.)

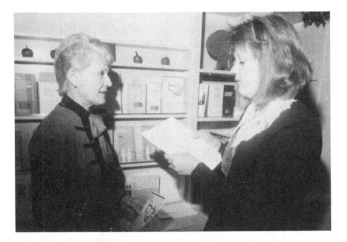

Walking Comes to the Malls—Elaine discusses literature offered to fitness walkers by A Measure Of Wellness, a clinic operating in a Southern California mall. The clinic provides blood pressure testing, books, pamphlets, films and a variety of fitness walks, including regular walks within the temperature-controlled mall.

Wellness Walk—A Measure Of Wellness has arranged with the management of the Courtyard Mall in Southern California to have the distances marked off within the temperature-controlled mall, making it much easier for fitness walkers to compute time, effort *and* distance.

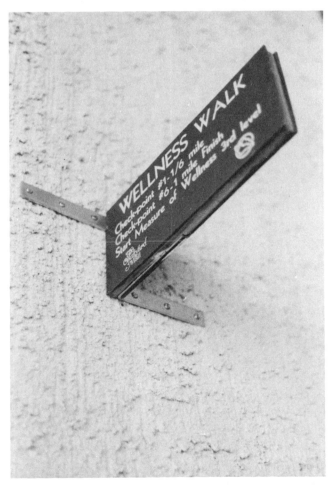

Allow some of your creativity to take hold. You'll be very pleasantly surprised at the results. And you'll never get bored.

Alone and Together

The lyrics to one song that was popular in the '60s claimed that "You'll never walk alone." To balance that sentiment, there is the saying that some people march (walk) to their own drummer—a drummer that the rest of us do not hear.

The question of whether you should consider walking alone or with one or more people is an important consideration. Let's briefly look at the pros and cons of both sides of the question:

Walking Alone

Pros: You can walk whenever and wherever you want. You can walk at a speed that is both comfortable and right for you without consideration of another person's pace (a pace that might not reap you maximum benefits). Walking alone frequently stimulates good feelings, simplifies complex and sticky issues in your mind, promotes solutions, and helps you to get in better touch with yourself.

Cons: For some, walking alone can be boring; that boredom can serve to undermine continuing in the activity. If you are not a person who is used to doing things independently, the prospects of engaging in a walking program alone can be overwhelming and can often undermine the resolve not just to stick with it, but to get it going in the first place. In some areas, it is not safe to walk alone. Some people like to talk while they walk, and society seems to frown on a person talking to him- or herself.

Walking Together

Pros: Walking with others provides good company and camaraderie, elements that usually encourage a person to stick with an activity. Other walkers can—and usually do—provide motivation to keep with a program; people who walk together regularly are the best coaches and cheerleaders in the world for each other. When you have a friend or several friends who walk with you, they are always willing to offer support when you feel down or uninspired. Walking with one or more friends establishes a time in each day when you can plan your walking without having to come up with your own plan. There is safety in numbers.

Cons: When you walk with others, you must walk at the speed of the slowest or weakest member of the group. This could undermine the benefits of the walk because the pace is not raising your pulse rate high enough. You are required to regulate your day to accommodate the time when the group goes out for its walk. A group frequently spends a great deal of talking while walking, which can tend to be a distraction from the object of the exercise.

As you can see, there is good and bad on each side of the coin.

Perhaps the perfect solution is to do a combination of both: walk with one or more friends on your "easy" days when performance is not your paramount objective. But reserve your "hard" days for yourself.

I personally enjoy walking both ways.

But, because of the hectic schedule that I frequently enjoy, my best walking experiences are often my solitary walks. The benefits I find from walking alone are these:

1. I learn to depend on myself and have a heightened sense of self-sufficiency. Although there is a certain feeling of shared power in walking with a group, I derive a tremendous feeling of well-being when I walk alone. It gets me more in touch with my own body, with how I move and—more importantly—with why I move. There are no conversational distractions, and as a result, I can feel the power flowing from the road up through my legs. It infuses me and refills my fuel tanks.

2. I feel very much that it is *my* walk, at my pace, according to my schedule. I feel beholden to no one. If my schedule for that day calls for 45 minutes of walking, I can set my resolve and *go!*

3. I love the occasional solitude a walk alone provides. It is great therapy against the increasingly complex world we live in and gives you an opportunity to get to know a person you perhaps have been putting off getting to know for years: yourself. I know several people who are terrified and have a huge fear of being alone. This is not a

healthy sign. We should all get to know ourselves better, to learn to be our own best friend. And what better way than to take yourself out for a long, solitary walk? It is a lot better than getting to know yourself through your fears in a lonely house or room. If you are one of those people who needs to have someone around all the time, try walking alone. You may find a side of yourself you've been supressing too long.

4. Although I go alone on many of my walks, I never find that I am lonely. When I walk alone, I am in control and I can plan my goals for that day. Also, I can take whatever tangents I want from my planned course. For instance, if I happen to see flowers or trees blooming on a hillside, I can deviate from my planned course and walk past them without consulting anyone. By the same token, if I find a lovely side road I've never walked before, I can head off down that road. Walt Whitman knew what he was talking about when he spoke of the freedom of the open road.

The Cautious Walker

It is not always in your best interest, however, to walk alone. The first commandment of the cautious walker is to avoid dangerous situations. Besides inclement weather, people, automobiles and dogs are pretty much the only sources of danger a walker faces. Let's take a look at them.

1. . . . People. There are some sections of the larger cities that are not only unsafe to pass through on foot but are also pretty chancy even in a motor vehicle. If you must walk through or near neighborhoods that you feel are dangerous, don't ever do so alone. Avoid it or walk with a friend, or preferably with a group of friends. Walking in a group offers some degree of protection. Most cities offer reduced rates on public transportation for the more mature citizens, and it is often worth the price of a ride to go to one of the city's parks where there are paths and roads designed for walkers. In New York's Central Park and San Francisco's Golden Gate Park, some of the roadways are blocked off over weekends to accommodate walkers, runners, skaters, and bicyclists. If your local park does not provide a safe place to walk, there is no reason you can't get together with a few friends and take your case to city hall.

When you find that you must walk alone, even if it is in seemingly safe neighborhoods, walk with authority. Just like in the animal kingdom, predators will be attracted to an animal that looks like prey. Don't walk in a furtive way that advertises you as a potential victim. Walk with confidence and authority and a sense of purpose. Make your strides meaningful and strong. And of course, do not walk wearing jewelry or other items of value that will attract someone of unsavory character to you.

And when you leave the house to go walking, always remember to tell someone where you are going and when you plan to be back. And get in the habit of carrying enough coins to make an emergency phone call should you run into trouble. Most warm-up outfits have a zippered pocket. There are also Velcro type wrist-bands with little change pockets in them that are made for walkers and runners. You can also get little pockets that attach to your shoelaces. Remember the Scouts' motto: be prepared.

You may also want to get into the habit of walking with a walking stick or cane. Walking sticks are very common in Europe and can be nice company as you swing them in rhythm to your walking. Walking sticks and other similar devices such as an umbrella, golf club or a simple telescoping automobile radio antenna can be effective deterrants to trouble.

Many people feel that carrying a can of Mace is the answer. Since Mace is considered a weapon in many states, you'll want to check into the laws that are in effect in your area. You'll also want to take a class in the use of Mace if you feel it is necessary to your peace of mind. Police report that people who carry Mace frequently don't know how to use it, and sometimes end up Macing themselves when the time for action comes. And because Mace is considered by some jurisdictions as a weapon, carrying a can without a license constitutes carrying a concealed weapon. If you are *that* apprehensive about taking your walk, either change locales or consult your local police department for advice.

2. . . . **Automobiles**. In certain suburban areas, and even in some hillside neighborhoods, as well as in the city, no considerations were made for pedestrians. These locales are devoid of sidewalks and people wanting to walk there had best be prepared to deal with motorists and their fumes, drainage ditches, unattended brush, discarded beer cans and the like. If there are dangerous stretches of roadway that feature inadequate provisions for pedestrians, no sense in taking any chances. Walk elsewhere.

3. . . . **Dogs**. And then there is "man's best friend," the dog. An unrestrained dog can be detrimental to a walker. Some dogs have a strong interest in biting while others are interested in playing or jumping on a walker to get affection.

When we lived in the Hollywood hills, almost everyone had dogs in their yards. As I took my walk each morning, I could tell the houses that had dogs because they all barked as I passed by. Each one wanted to protect its territory. Once in a while a dog would get out and it was a problem to know whether the dog was friend or foe. Having been bitten by a dog when I was a child, I tend to be very cautious, but having had dogs all my life, I never let them get the upper hand—or any hand, for that matter. I do not make quick moves, I am not afraid, and I give them a command to sit or stay or just say, "Go home!" in a firm voice. Don't ever turn or run from a dog; the dog may take that as a signal that you are prey and it will act accordingly. Speak in a voice of authority, stand your ground and give it a command to sit, stay or go home. Dogs sense if you are afraid. And again, a device such as a walking stick will often come in handy in discouraging a dog from bothering you.

Try to avoid neighborhoods where dogs are prevalent, and if you are bothered by a dog, don't suffer in silence; talk first to the dog's owner and, if you are unable to get in touch with the owner, tell the authorities. There are leash laws in most towns and cities, and the local animal control agent will be happy to see they are enforced.

This section merely points out the potential dangers that a walker can face. Most walkers will put literally thousands of miles on their walking shoes without encountering any dangers. In fact, they encounter nothing on their walks but enjoyment; however, it is always best to be a little bit more cautious than not. A little well-placed caution goes a long way toward keeping you safe and sound.

Weather Watch

A relatively healthy person can walk in virtually any climate if certain precautions are taken relative to clothing, pace and self-evaluation. The exceptions to this statement would be centered more on surface conditions than on weather. For instance, walking on an icy or sleet-covered sidewalk is dangerous no matter how fit and healthy a person is.

There are two major weather conditions that should be approached with caution: extreme heat (and/or humidity) and extreme cold.

In extremely hot weather conditions, even the body lying on a chaise lounge next to a swimming pool is undergoing certain kinds of physical pressure or stress. Add humidity and the situation is compounded.

Hot weather causes the human body to work hard at cooling itself. Although the human cooling systems are a marvel of biological engineering, they do not accomplish their goals of cooling without energy being expended by the body. Just as cities caught in the grip of a heat wave experience electrical brown-outs when too many air conditioners place an excessive demand on the power sources, so it is with the human body. The body becomes much less efficient during the heat because so much of its energies are already being taxed to stay at normal body temperature.

Throw in humidity (which inhibits the body's ability to cool by sending perspiration to the surface of the skin to have it evaporated into the surrounding air), and the exertion involved can be quite exaggerated.

It is always a good rule of thumb that when the weather conditions go above 80/80 (80 degrees and 80% humidity), strenuous exercise for those above 50 years of age should be curtailed in consideration of the tremendous demands placed upon the body to both cool itself and to perform exercise at the same time.

During periods of extreme heat and/or humidity, you can get around the problem by exercising very early in the morning or in the early evening, when the sun is either not out or is low on the horizon. Even though the air temperature may be high at those times of the day, there is no additional danger present from the sun's radiant heat beating on your body.

If you do exercise during the day in a climate that is hot but low in humidity, it is important to wear lightweight, light-colored, loose-fitting, breathable clothes to help reflect the sun's rays. A whitish-toned reflective hat is also important. This is also an effective way to help the body maintain its cool.

In extreme circumstances, where the temperature and humidity are over 80, why not consider doing your walking in the nearest body of water? When it is extremely hot, I love to get into a pool up to my shoulders, walk around, and then do some water exercises. The pool water keeps my skin cooled and the resistance of the water can provide quite a workout in a fraction of the time. (We'll discuss this method in more detail in the next section.)

The ideal weather conditions are at the nearby enclosed shopping mall. The mall temperatures are usually very agreeable.

The most important caution, however, is to drink plenty of water. Sip water all day long. And try to go through a minimum of two quarts per day. Remember that the sensation of thirst means you are well behind in keeping up with your body's water needs.

The other weather extreme is cold.

As long as you are dressed properly, cold weather should never be a problem—unless there are accompanying bad footing conditions.

If you dress in layers, you'll find that once you have begun walking, your body will generate warmth. It is nature's own little furnace. Dressing in layers allows some of the body's warm air to get trapped between the layers, which serves as insulation. It also provides easy temperature control. As your body warms up, you can cool down a bit by removing your outer jacket and tying it around your hips by the sleeves. Then, if you begin to cool down unexpectedly, just slip the jacket on again.

You should always cover your head with some type of warm headgear. A woolen ski hat is excellent. In cold weather, the body loses approximately half of its heat through the head. Covering the head holds in a good deal of precious body heat.

Also consider wearing a light turtleneck shirt as your first garment. The turtleneck keeps the major arteries in the neck warm, and when they are warm, you feel warmer and more comfortable. Also, if it becomes warm during your walk, turtlenecks can be turned down to reveal part of the neck, which serves as an almost instant cooling mechanism.

Be certain to wear gloves of some sort, also. Mittens are best because they provide more warmth than gloves with fingers: the body warmth coming from your fingers is exchanged in mittens, rather than absorbed by the material of the gloves.

In extremely cold weather, people begin to worry about taking in deep breaths of air. The body makes provisions to warm the air before it hits the lungs, but the sensation of the extremely cold air being sucked into the throat can be disconcerting. Consider wearing a ski mask over your head. The material of the mask will help warm the air before it enters your mouth. This protection is especially important when it is cold *and* windy. The wind-chill factor can make a cold day almost unbearable.

I remember many a winter day trudging across campus at the University of Minnesota with a scarf over my face so all you could see were my eyes. Sometimes the temperature would go down as low as 40 or 50 below. Brrrrrrr.

Also, remember that while you are exercising with your three layers of clothing, your ski mask and your mittens (and hopefully your leather walking shoes), your body is producing perspiration. The perspiration comes in the form of very small droplets of moisture. But even on cold days, perspiration is being formed to help regulate the body's temperature. The moisture lost in the process of temperature control should be replaced. Even during the middle of winter, it is wise to drink about two quarts of water a day. Don't let the cold weather fool you into thinking otherwise.

Surface Conditions

At one time, before paved roads, our ancestors walked on country roads of dirt and city streets that were also dirt. In order to avoid the mud that formed on a city street during a rainstorm, wooden sidewalks were added, and eventually the solution of paving the streets came about. Today, we tend to walk primarily on concrete sidewalks or asphalt pavement when we are out of doors.

Both concrete and asphalt are very hard surfaces (although concrete is several times harder than asphalt). It is very fortunate that the science of making good walking shoes has progressed to the point it has, or there would be more than the 70% of the population who experience some sort of foot problems.

Many foot problems, however, are caused by years—even decades—of wearing improper shoes. If the shoe does *not* support the foot properly, it can actually deform the foot by chronically forcing it into unnatural angles.

Is it any wonder, then, that by the time the human foot gets to be 50-plus, it is crying for relief? Thank goodness for the Running Revolution in the '70s and the Walking Revolution in the '80s; it made running and walking shoes more comfortable, more fashionable, and our feet much happier.

The well-made walking shoe is the walker's first defense against different kinds of surfaces.

Besides sidewalks, bike, and asphalt paths being hard on the feet, many natural surfaces can be difficult for the walker, especially eroded dirt and rocky paths. When walking in the sand, downhill, or on a bridle path layered with redwood chips, be aware that these surfaces put more demands on the legs and feet. For instance, if you walk uphill you are using different muscles than you would be walking downhill or walking in the sand. In sand walking, the toes work harder to grip and additional tension is placed on the Achilles tendon and calf. So if you do change your terrain, it is important to be mindful of the fact that in doing so you are using different muscles; therefore, you must start out easy.

I like to vary the kinds of walking surfaces because it gives my muscles a challenge (as long as I don't overdo it). I tend to avoid hiking on hazardous trails and roads that are heavily traveled by automobiles.

Have you ever walked in the water? If so, remember having to put forth more effort in order to walk? This is another way of adding variety to your walking program. The water gives resistance, challenging your muscles so that they can become stronger.

If you have access to a pool, try walking across the lower end of it, back and forth. Take short strides and then long strides. I even lift my knees as high as possible (similar to a majorette or a drum major marching in a parade). I'd like to suggest, too, that while in the water you can do all the lower body exercises suggested in Chapter 6. I happen to like to swim a few laps, do a little water workout in the lower end of the pool and then do a few more laps. For those of you who don't swim, you can stand in the water, shoulder-height, and simulate the swimming stroke. If you are in a hot tub, bend your knees (squatting position) so that your shoulders are in the water and cup your hand so that you can pull the water back as you use the swimming movement. The resistance of the water gives you a great workout.

Water walking and water exercises also help combat injuries because the buoyancy of the water helps to take the strain off the muscles and joints while still providing resistance and a good workout.

Most of my walking, however, is still done on the conventional surfaces all of us face every day: concrete sidewalks and asphalt roads. It's difficult to escape them.

You can make both surfaces your friends, though, by using good walking shoes to protect the foot from impact, and by progressing with your walking program at a rate that allows your joints and ligaments to become fit simultaneously with your lungs. And that's what my programs will build upon, as you'll see over the next several chapters.

Chapter 5

Vital Signs

"The palms of your hands will thicken,
The skin of your cheek will tan,
You'll go ragged and weary and swarthy,
But you'll walk like a man"
"Do You Hear the Wind?"
—Hamlin Garland

Think of this chapter in the same way you would think of the instrument panel of your car. The instrument panel tells you what various systems of the car are doing. What is the temperature of the fluid in the cooling system? How much gasoline is in the tank? How many miles traveled on the trip odometer? Is the battery being charged properly?

This chapter will serve to keep you abreast of what your body is doing at the beginning of your walking program, and all through it. At the same time, it will provide an ongoing record of your preventive maintenance.

These are the five measurements that are of primary concern. They are measurements of progress and speed indicators. Once you know these, you will not have to rely on subjective perceptions.

1. . . . **Resting Pulse Rate.** Your pulse rate functions as the tachometer of your body's motor. It shows you a good—and efficient—range in which to do your walking so that you will gain physical benefits, but will not overdo it. Just how to figure out your safe range of exercise we will discuss when we reach that section. Your resting pulse rate corresponds to what an automobile is doing when the motor is idling. The best time to take your resting pulse rate is first thing in the morning, before

you get out of bed. Set a watch with a second hand on your bedside table; also have a pad and pencil beside the watch. When you wake up, take your pulse rate either at your wrist or at your neck. Count your pulse for 15 seconds and then simply multiply by four. Jot down your pulse rate next to the date on your pad of paper. Normally, the pulse rate falls somewhere between 50 and 90 beats per minute. Over a period of months on my walking program, you should be able to see your resting pulse rate drop by perhaps 10 beats or more. This indicates that your heart is doing its job more efficiently. If your pulse rate is occasionally elevated, don't become concerned. This can occur occasionally if you have a period of stress or if you have not fully recovered from a physical effort from the day before. If you chart your resting pulse rate daily, you should begin to see a pattern that varies very little. On the charts that follow, we'll plot it every three months, where the changes will show up much more dramatically.

2. . . . **Blood Pressure**. The blood pressure is a very good indicator of health: both good and bad. High blood pressure (hypertension) is a warning sign that something is wrong. Even with all the marvelous scientific research we have these days, the cause of most high blood pressure is un-

known, but we do know that many factors contribute to it. We know, too, that it is more likely present in people who have certain physical characteristics and certain habits. An obese person is more likely to have higher blood pressure and so is a person who smokes cigarettes. Stress is also a factor. Blood pressure is the force that is exerted against the sides of the arteries by the blood as it is pumped through the body. If there is an inflexibility of the arteries, if they are clogged with plaque, or if the blood is pumped with unusually high force, the blood pressure is going to be higher. Blood pressure, as you probably already know, is measured in two numbers, one over the other. The first number is the systolic pressure, which is the period during which the heart contracts and first sends the pressure through the arteries. The second number measures the diastolic pressure, which is the period when the heart is relaxed and fills with blood; this period is marked by a drop in pressure in the arteries. The two numbers, then,

indicate the highest and lowest pressures on the artery walls. For the average 20-year-old, the measurement is usually 120 over 80. As we age, the blood pressure inches upwards. With a regular program of modest exercise, like walking, you should see your blood pressure either stabilize or begin to drop. Once again, we will be plotting it every three months. You can regularly have your blood pressure taken quickly and easily in a variety of ways: during regular check-ups by your doctor, in shopping malls, as an ongoing service in walk-in clinics, etc., or you can choose to purchase your own blood pressure cuff (sphygmomanometer).

3. . . . **Serum Cholesterol**. There has been plenty written in the newspapers and magazines over the past few years about the effects of too much cholesterol in the diet. Cholesterol tends to clog the arteries, which in turn causes high blood pressure and can ultimately starve the heart of much-needed oxygen and nutrients. More heart disease is caused by clogged arteries than by a

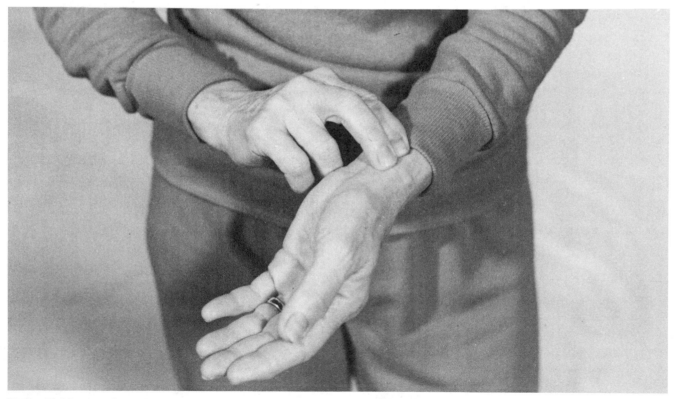

Pulse-Taking at the Wrist—The most common method of taking the pulse is to use the wrist. Find the pulse on the underside of the wrist and touch it lightly. The pulse rate is the body's tachometer. It is an integral monitor of every exercise program.

weak heart. The more cholesterol we consume, the faster and more thoroughly the arteries will be clogged and the higher our risk of heart problems.

When I was a young girl living in Minneapolis, our evening meal most always consisted of meat, potatoes, vegetables and cake or pie for dessert. I can remember washing dishes, especially the pots and pans. The pots in which the meat was cooked were always filled with gooey fat. By the time dinner was over, the fat had hardened, so I would take hot water and soap to melt it and then pour it down the drain. Frequently, over a period of time, the fat would clog the drain. So it is with our arteries. Fat likes to cling to our artery walls, and if we do not move it along through good nutrition and exercise, it clogs our arteries to the point the blood has trouble getting through. Then when one little clot comes along, it can plug up the artery and *Poof*—a heart attack or stroke.

By exercising and cutting down on our intake of cholesterol, we can lower it. The number recorded in the space provided in the following chart will come from a simple blood test. The test can be retaken every three months at a hospital, clinic, or a health/fitness facility. These days the test is quick, simple and accurate. The number you will receive is in milligrams of cholesterol in about every three and one-half ounces of blood. A number between 200 and 220 is considered normal; above 220 is cause for concern, because it is above the 220 where most heart attacks occur; a number below 200 is very desirable.

4. . . . **Body Fat**. Thank goodness we have moved away from the days when we thought that someone reed-thin was at the height of fashion and the height of physical perfection. These days, the ideal is better muscled and defined: more ideally human by Greek standards than by starvation standards. The human body needs some fat. However, the fat should be in our bodies, not *on* our

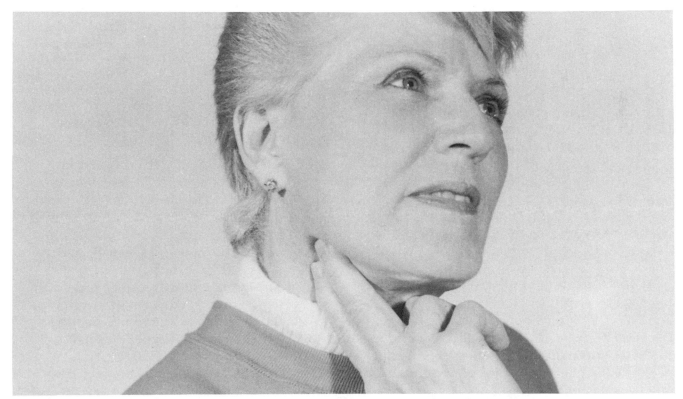

Pulse-Taking at the Neck—The pulse can also be taken at the neck. Remember that in order to feel the pulse accurately, once the artery is found, it should not be pressed down. This will inhibit the proper passage of blood and will throw off your count. Touch the pulse just enough so that you can feel it accurately.

bodies. Dietary fat is essential for some human functions, such as energy and growth, assimilating fat-soluble vitamins and lubricating the skin and other tissue. The *Mayo Clinic Health Letter* states, in an article on dietary fat, "Dietary fat carries vitamins A, D, E and K, and supplies energy as well as fatty acids essential to proper nutrition." And it goes on to say, "We all need fat in our diet, but most of us get too much."

Too much fat causes a whole battery of life-threatening problems, from high blood pressure and heart disease to diabetes. So try to cut back on your fat intake. Check to see if you're indulging in too many dairy products, fatty meats, fried foods, snacks and desserts. Remember, a little may be okay, but too much is always too much.

If one apple a day is good for you, you wouldn't eat a hundred, would you? Therefore, we go back to what we were saying in Chapter 3: everything in moderation.

Body fat can be measured in a variety of ways: body fat calipers, sending low-grade electrical impulses through the body, immersion in a water tank. Most hospitals, some health clubs and sports medicine departments of colleges and universities offer body fat testing by calipers. It is a good idea to have a reading of your body fat content. But for the sake of consistency of these readings, it would be best to decide on what type of measuring device you'll adopt and then stick with it throughout your program. Males should strive for less than 15% body fat, while women should strive for less than 22%.

5. . . . **Body Weight**. Total body weight is what you get when you step on the bathroom scale. For a number of reasons, body weight is not a good guide to whether or not you are fit and healthy. Among those reasons: different people have different body structures and different size bones and therefore a person who is the same height as the next person may actually be leaner although he or she weights more; upon the initiation of a fitness program, it is very common for a person to add weight as muscle mass (which weighs more but consumes less space than fat) increases and fat stores (which weigh less but consume more space) decrease. For instance, your weight may not have changed much since high school or college, but your waistline has increased considerably due to lack of exercise. This is due to the fact that muscle tone has decreased while fat deposits have increased. Even though you weigh the same you measure in larger and softer. I include the place to record total body weight in the charts following merely as a baseline measurement that is traditional but not critical. It is much less important than the measurement of body fat.

You can use the following charts to record your measurements every three months for up to three years and three months. At the end of the charts there is an additional page that does not feature any year-and-month designations at the top so that you can continue beyond the three years. This additional page can be photocopied, filled in and inserted in your book as needed.

The first entry is keyed to where you are now. Take the time to get the measurements when embarking on your walking program, and jot them down. Take your resting pulse rate and body weight. A visit to your doctor can provide blood pressure, serum cholesterol and body fat. Then get ready to chart your progress to fitness and health. It's one report card you'll be very happy to show around.

Gauging Your Working Heart Rate (WHR)

Almost every high-performance car comes equipped with a tachometer. The tachometer is a device that monitors the revolutions of the automobile's motor. As a motor's revolutions per minute build, the motor approaches its maximum horsepower or performance. When the maximum horsepower is reached, the power curve begins to drop off and any additional revolutions per minute will not improve the motor's power. In fact, there is a redline on the tachometer to warn you that any additional rpms will actually begin to damage the motor.

The human heart works very much like the automobile's motor. Instead of revolutions per minute, it produces beats per minute. Instead of a tachometer, the human being has a pulse that indicates the number of beats per minute the heart is producing.

Like the automobile engine, the heart has a resting rate (comparable to a motor's idle). It has a power curve that climbs as more demand is placed upon it, it has a point where it is working at top performance, and it has a point beyond which any more beats can actually undermine the heart's efficiency.

It is essential that the 50 + walker knows these VIPs (Very Important Points).

We've already mentioned the Resting Pulse Rate that you should be taking before you get out of bed each morning. The RPR (Resting Pulse Rate) gives you a reading of how efficient your heart is at rest. As you become more fit and healthier, the RPR will begin to drop until it settles in at a very comfortable number of beats per minute. The number will almost always be significantly lower than it was before you began exercising, because with exercise, your heart strengthens and is able to provide the necessary oxygen and nutrients with less effort. The RPR will likely drop some 10 points after a year of exercising, and in some cases may drop as much as 20 points.

At the other extreme of the heart's ability to beat is what we can call the MHR (Maximum Heart Rate). This corresponds with the motor's redline. At that point the heart could injure itself because it is pumping much too fast. You would never want to approach the MHR except under a doctor's supervision while undergoing a maximal stress test.

Somewhere in between these two extremes there is a range where your heart will beat efficiently because it is meeting its bodily needs caused by exercise. It is in this range that your heart becomes stronger and your blood circulatory system is improved. This is also the point where exercise of an aerobic nature is helping the body thrive. Because of the gradual degenerative processes of aging, this point is lower for a 50-year-old than it is for a 20-year-old. For the purposes of my walking program, we're going to refer to this range as the WHR—Working Heart Rate. The range will be from 60 to 80 percent of your theoretical MHR (Maximum Heart Rate).

Here's how you go about determining your WHR (Working Heart Rate):

1. Start with the number 220.

2. Subtract your age (let's use 60). That gives us 160.

3. Now take percentages of the 160 that correspond to 60%, 70% and 80%. They come out to the following:

60% = 96 beats per minute
70% = 112 beats per minute
80% = 128 beats per minute

These are the three numbers you need to know to get the maximum benefits out of this program. As you'll see in Chapter 8, a starter's program will begin with the 60% number. And from there, over a period of time, we'll gradually work up to 70% efforts and then ultimately to 80% efforts as we get into the more advanced levels of walking. When we get to 80%, efforts at 60 and 70% will be considered easy workout days. As I mentioned earlier, we won't be concentrating so much with distance, but more with time and work (as indicated by WHR). The distance you cover will merely be incidental. (Remember that in an automobile, the odometer—which measures the miles traveled—is much smaller on the dashboard than the speedometer and tachometer.)

This would be a good place to record your WHR. Why not see what your WHR should be? Fill in your beats per minute that correspond to your percentages according to your age:

> **My heart rate at 60% will be** _____ **beats per minute.**
> **My heart rate at 70% will be** _____ **beats per minute.**
> **My heart rate at 80% will be** _____ **beats per minute.**

You'll want to remember these three numbers, because they will serve as your tachometer for the entire program. If you have trouble remembering them, write them down on a slip of paper and carry them in your pocket. Or, write them down on a small piece of paper and Scotch tape it to the back of your wristwatch as a reminder. Then, if you forget, you can consult them very easily.

Remember that without these numbers, your program won't work. They are numbers that will keep you from going too fast—and, just as importantly, they'll keep you from going too slow!

VITAL SIGNS	START OF PROGRAM	3 MONTHS	6 MONTHS
RESTING PULSE RATE	bpm	bpm	bpm
BLOOD PRESSURE			
SERUM CHOLESTEROL	mg.	mg.	mg.
BODY FAT	%	%	%
BODY WEIGHT	lbs.	lbs.	lbs.
NOTES/ OBSERVATIONS			

9 MONTHS	1 YEAR	1 YEAR, 3 MONTHS	1 YEAR, 6 MONTHS
bpm	bpm	bpm	bpm
mg.	mg.	mg.	mg.
%	%	%	%
lbs.	lbs.	lbs.	lbs.

VITAL SIGNS

	1 YEAR, 9 MONTHS	2 YEARS	2 YEARS, 3 MONTHS
RESTING PULSE RATE	bpm	bpm	bpm
BLOOD PRESSURE			
SERUM CHOLESTEROL	mg.	mg.	mg.
BODY FAT	%	%	%
BODY WEIGHT	lbs.	lbs.	lbs.
NOTES/ OBSERVATIONS			

2 YEARS, 6 MONTHS	2 YEARS, 9 MONTHS	3 YEARS	3 YEARS, 3 MONTHS
bpm	bpm	bpm	bpm
mg.	mg.	mg.	mg.
%	%	%	%
lbs.	lbs.	lbs.	lbs.

VITAL SIGNS			
RESTING PULSE RATE	bpm	bpm	bpm
BLOOD PRESSURE			
SERUM CHOLESTEROL	mg.	mg.	mg.
BODY FAT	%	%	%
BODY WEIGHT	lbs.	lbs.	lbs.
NOTES/ OBSERVATIONS			

Chapter 6

Warm-Up/Cool-Down Exercises

*"Not to go back is somewhat to advance,
And men must walk, at least, before they dance."*

—Alexander Pope

I have a saying tacked up on my kitchen wall. "Don't put off until tomorrow what you can do today." I must confess that, at times, I am a procrastinator and tend to want to put things off. One such "thing" I think about putting off is my workouts. It's easy to find excuses like: "I'm too busy." "I'm on a deadline." "There just isn't enough time."

However, as I said in a previous chapter, we always seem to find the time to do the things we really want to do.

I soon realized that this "time excuse" was pretty feeble and that the problem was really me.

An example of that was this morning. I woke up later than usual and wrestled with myself thinking, "I'm on a deadline for this book. I'll do it tomorrow." But staring at that little reminder quote on the wall, the other side of me said, "Make time!"

Not only did I make time, but I did my warm-up and walk, a host of other exercises, and ended up cooling down by swimming and walking in the pool. I felt so refreshed, so exhilarated, and so proud of myself. Afterward I thought, "How senseless it was of me to want to put off this great feeling."

If you tend to want to procrastinate, think of the *results* you're putting off. It really helps to keep you on the ball.

I must admit, however, that there *was* a time in my life when I gave up. I just didn't care anymore.

I lost my beautiful 21-year-old red-headed daughter in an automobile accident and I was completely and totally devastated. A physically sound, vivacious, happy life was snuffed out in one day. We were so close that I felt I had been snuffed out, too. Months went by and I saw myself, literally, going to pot. Then one day I woke up to the fact that the less I did, the worse I felt, and Janet wouldn't be proud to see me this way. I gradually started taking long walks and in no time I began feeling much better physically. Jack encouraged me to put more effort into my walking by using his Dynastriding method. It wasn't long before I was back to my workouts and not only feeling better physically, but mentally as well.

We have all had adversities of one sort or another in our lives. But they are no reason to give up. I am reminded of the expression, "The only thing constant about life is change." We live in a changing world; our lives are constantly changing and our bodies are also changing. If we lead an inactive life, our bodies change to reflect that lifestyle.

By the same token, if we live an active life, our bodies change to display that particular way of life.

In his lectures, Jack often refers to all of us as "walking billboards." Think of yourself as a walking billboard and let's walk to build an attractive billboard. However, before we start our walk, let's do some warm-up exercises.

Why warm up before we walk? To avoid stiffness, soreness, and possible injury to the muscles, joints, tendons and ligaments. It also facilitates efficient movement. Think of a rusty old hinge. It creaks and groans until you keep moving it. The more you move it, the easier it moves.

By taking five minutes to warm up before you walk, you'll prolong your ability to exercise while also making your Dynastriding more fluid and effortless.

What follows are some of my warm-up exercises that I'd like you to try. They can be done alone, either indoors or outdoors, or with a group. Whichever way you do them, make a habit of doing them. Consistency is the key. The time of day is up to you. Don't leave home without them.

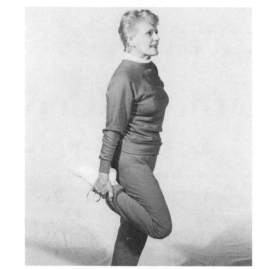

Knee and Thigh Stretch—Balance yourself against a wall, a chair, or a tree with your left hand. Grasp your right ankle with your left hand and pull up to stretch thigh muscle. Repeat on left leg. Repeat 5 times per leg.

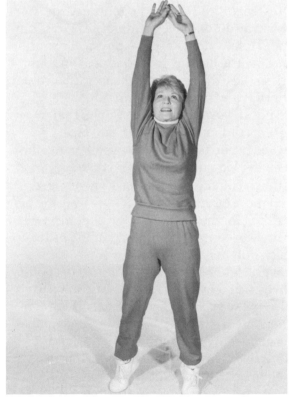

The Sky Stretch—Spread feet shoulder-width apart. Now, lift your arms over your head, palms up, fingers touching. Stretch as if you were trying to touch the ceiling or the sky. Count to 10.

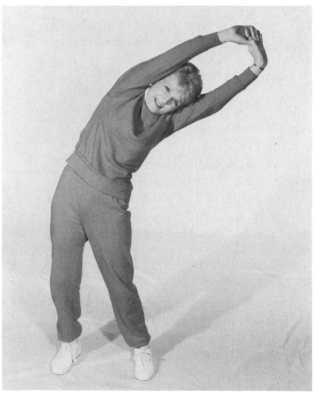

The Side-to-Side Stretch—Begin just as you would the Sky Stretch. While reaching for the sky, keep the feet planted solidly on the earth. Now, bend at the waist from side to side. Do this one to a count of 10 to each side: 1 left, 1 right, 2 left, 2 right, etc.

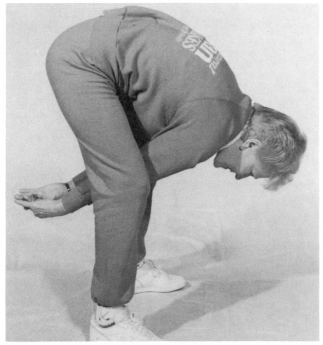

Through the Legs Stretch—Plant your feet shoulder-width apart. Bend forward at the waist, knees bent slightly to take the strain off the back. Bring the hands through the legs, attempting to touch the floor and wall behind you. Hold for a count of 10.

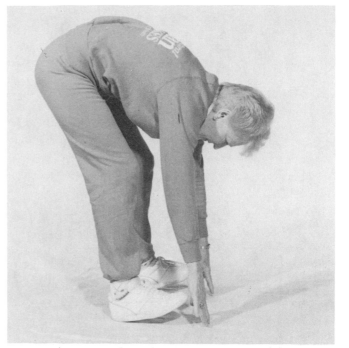

Hamstring Stretch—Place your feet shoulder-width apart. Bend forward at the waist, knees bent slightly. Allow your hands to drop down in front of your feet, as though trying to touch the floor. Now, lift the toes off the floor. Hold for a count of 2. Feel those hamstrings stretch!

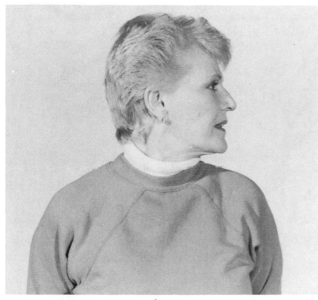

Side-to-Side Neck Conditioner—Move your head from side to side as far as you can without exerting undue force. Repeat it to the left and then the right. Don't move your shoulders. Try to repeat this one 10 times.

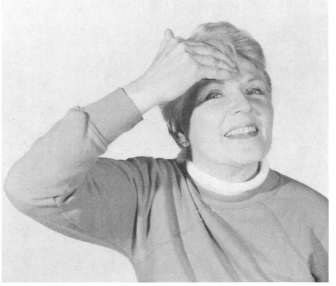

Up-and-Down Neck Conditioner—Lift your head up and look at the ceiling, then bring your head down, attempting to place your chin on your chest. When you become stronger, use your hand to offer resistance. This exercise (along with the previous exercise) helps condition the front, back and sides of the neck, and brings a good blood supply to the extremities. Do this one 10 times.

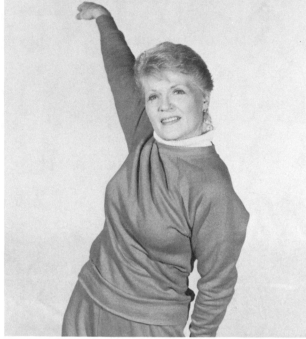

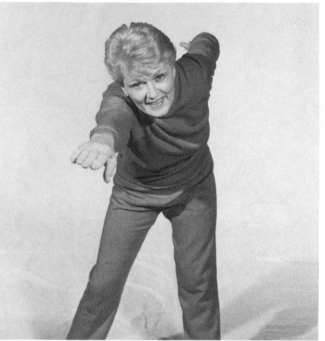

Swimming Motion: BACKSTROKE—Plant your feet shoulder-width apart. Lift your arm up and stroke it back as in the backstroke. Alternate arms, just as though you were really in a pool. This one helps round shoulders, and is good for posture in general. Go to a count of 20 on this one, 10 counts on each side.

Swimming Motion: CRAWL—Place your feet shoulder-width apart. Bend forward at the waist, with bent knees. Pretend you're doing the crawl: bring your right arm up over your ear and reach forward, your left arm going back. Alternate. This one helps the shoulders, back of arms and sides of the waist. Go to a count of 20, 10 counts on each side.

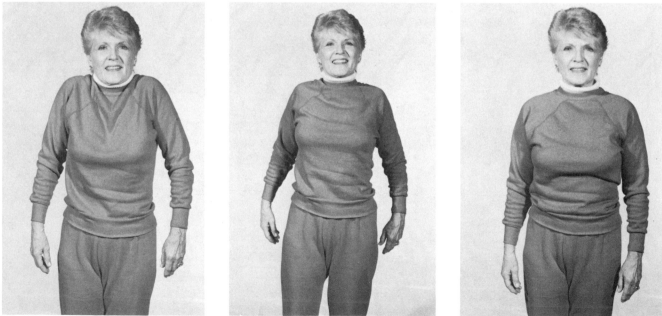

Shoulder Shrugs—Stand straight, feet shoulder-width apart. Relax your shoulders. Now, bring your shoulders up toward your ears, hold for a count of 3, then roll your shoulders back toward your back, hold for a count of 3, then return to starting position. This one is terrific for those of you who suffer from tension in the neck and shoulders.

52

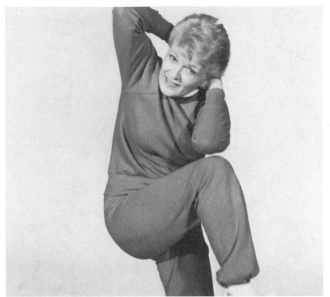

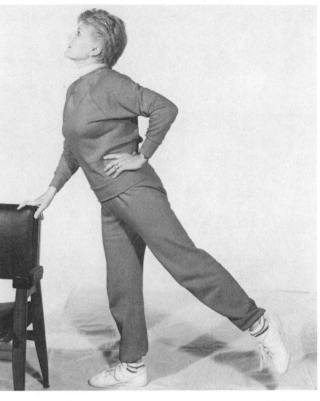

Knee into Chest—Stand erect with your feet shoulder-width apart. With your hands behind your head, bring the right knee up and try to touch the left elbow. Alternate. Do 5 on each leg. Remember to bring the leg up to the elbow; don't move the elbow down to the knee.

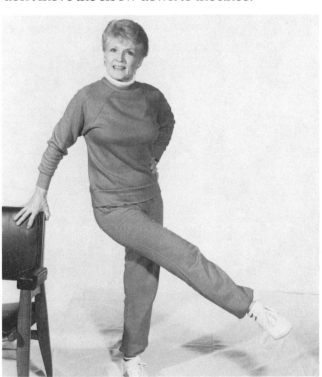

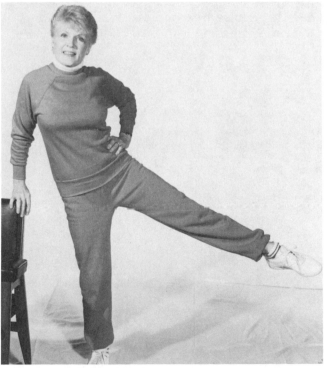

Leg Extensions—This one involves three separate motions. Begin by standing erect with your feet shoulder-width apart, one hand on a hip, the other resting on a chair back for support. Now, point your toe, extend right leg to the back as far as possible (hold for count of 5); then, out to the side as far as possible (hold for count of 5). Now flex foot (turn toes upward) and cross the same leg (right) over in front of opposite leg (hold for count of 5). Repeat on other leg. Go through this routine 10 times on each leg.

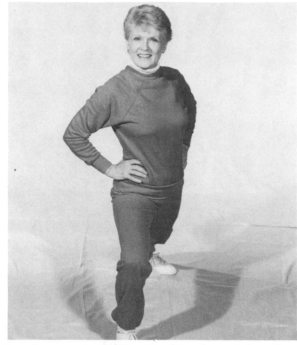 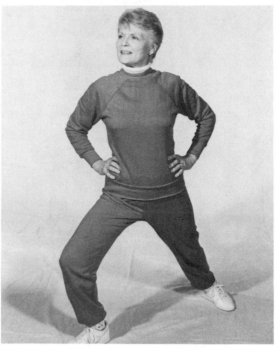

Leg Lunges to the Front—Stand erect, hands on hips (or on a chair for balance). Lunge forward similar to a fencing pose. Step back and lunge forward on the opposite leg. Do 5 lunges on each leg. These are wonderful for keeping the hips and thighs tight and firm.

Leg Lunges to the Side—Stand erect, hands on hips (or on a chair for balance). Lunge to the right with the right leg, step back and lunge to the left with the left leg. Do this one 5 times on each leg. This works the muscles from a different angle than the previous exercise.

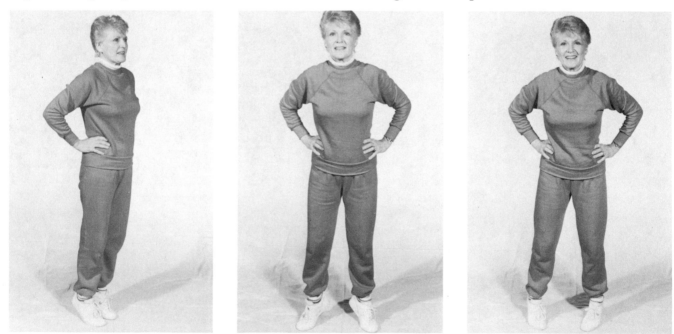

Toe Raises—Stand erect, with your feet in a comfortable position. Raise yourself up on your toes for a count of 2, and then lower yourself back to your starting position. Repeat 20 times. Now, for a variation, point your toes outwards away from your body, and raise yourself on your toes and then lower yourself. Repeat 20 times. For the third variation, stand pigeon-toed, raise and lower yourself 20 times. This really strengthens the legs and is terrific for increasing flexibility in the calf of the lower legs.

54

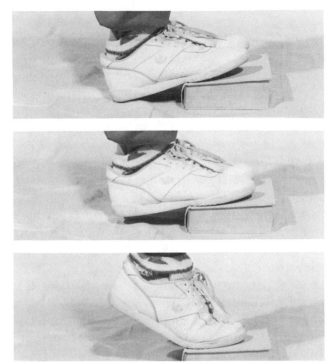

Toe Raises, Method 2—Holding onto a chair for balance, use a sturdy book or a block or wood, place your toes on the edge. Now, lower your heels to the floor, hold for a count of 2, then lift your heels up off the floor as high as you can, trying to stand on your toes for a count of 2.

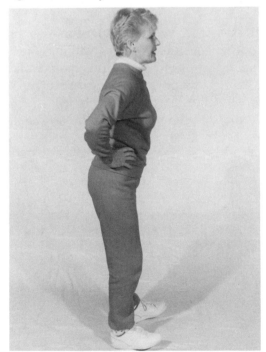

Heel Raises—Raise the toes up, weight on the heels. Hold for a count of 2. Repeat 10 times. This one is good for the tibialis muscle (next to your shinbone).

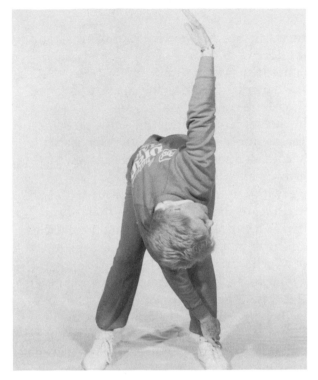

Windmill Stretch—Bend over at the waist. Try to touch the left hand to the ceiling while grasping the left ankle with the right hand. Bend knees slightly to take strain off back. Now alternate, reaching the right hand to the ceiling while grasping the right ankle with the left hand. Repeat 10 times to each side. You're finished, and you're ready to Dynastride!

The All-Important Cool-Down Exercises

The number of people who exercise and do not bother to cool-down is startling. Perhaps they are on such a high from their exercising that the cool-down phase seems totally unnecessary. Cool-down exercises gradually bring your body down from its exercising state to a near-resting state. They allow your blood flow to gradually return to normal, your breathing to come back to normal, all of your body systems to cool down to neutral.

How important are cool-down exercises? I'd like to include here a newspaper column on cool-down that my writing partner, Richard Benyo, wrote. He is the fitness columnist for the San Francisco *Chronicle*, and former executive editor of *Runner's World* Magazine. Here is the column:

There are three essential elements of any workout: the warm-up, the workout routine itself, and the cool-down.

Without the workout routine as the heart, there's no need to warm up or cool down; its importance as the keystone goes without saying.

In the question of whether the warm-up or the cool-down is more important, most exercisers, even hard-core ones, would quickly answer that the warm-up should predominate.

It is very important, after all, to warm up the muscles that are about to be used so that they are stretched and supple. By warming up the muscles before a workout, you reduce the chance of injury.

All of which is correct, of course.

In perspective, however, the cool-down is much more important than the warm-up, yet many people go so far as to completely ignore cool-down. They stop their exercise and stand around chatting with a friend, or they stop their exercise and immediately head for the showers.

Such an abrupt end to vigorous exercise can not only be ill-advised, it can be fatal.

Dr. Ken Cooper, father of aerobics, did a significant amount of research into the importance of the cool-down period subsequent to the death of Jim Fixx. "In short," Cooper says, "anyone who stops vigorous exercise abruptly is endangering his heart—and may be flirting with sudden death. The circulatory system in a sense goes 'out of balance' as the flow of blood slows down faster than the beating of the heart.

"If you stop and stand still without reducing the level of your activity step-by-step, your blood pressure will drop. But the natural stimulants from the adrenal glands keep the heart beating at a high and inefficient rate. As a result, not enough blood gets to the heart, and ischemia of the heart, involving a lack of blood to the heart tissue, may result. If there is too little blood that gets through to the heart, sudden death may occur."

Cooper theorizes that this factor may have contributed to the death of Jim Fixx. Fixx stopped immediately following a run on a hot day. He collapsed along the side of the road, propped against a small hillside. Cooper additionally theorizes that had Fixx fallen prone, it would have allowed blood to flow to the heart.

At the cessation of virtually any exercise, the best thing you can do to cool down is to walk.

If you want to compare notes on the workout with your training partner, you can compare them while walking off the workout. But don't stand in one place and compare notes. And don't ever just outright stop the exercise and stand around or sit down.

Make life easy on your heart's recovery. Give your heart a chance to gradually mellow out after you've asked it to do so much on your behalf.

*   *   *

Richard's advice to walk after vigorous exercise is very good. Even after vigorous walking, the first step in cooling down is to slow down your walking pace to a gentle, leisurely walk or stroll. If you can do this for five minutes, that's excellent.

Then, make it a point to do the following cool-down exercise routine.

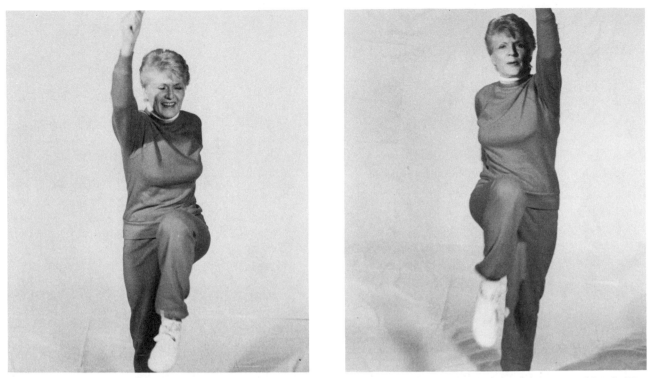

Marching—To begin the cool-down sequence, march in place, picking the knees up nice and high like a drum major or a majorette. Do this one for a total count of 20.

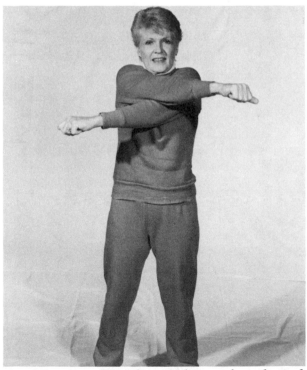

Arm Crosses—Standing with your feet planted shoulder-width apart, hold your arms out to the sides, parallel to the floor, while making a tight fist. Do not bend arms. Now, bring them in across your chest, and then swing them back out, looking up at the ceiling. Repeat this one 20 times.

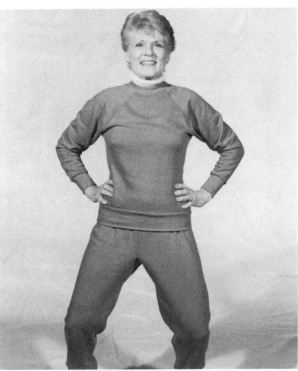

Half Squats—Stand erect, feet shoulder-width apart, bend your knees, lean back slightly trying to keep your shoulders behind your heels. Bend and straighten 3 times.

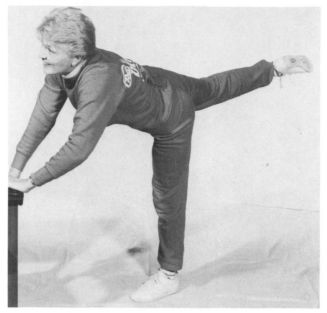

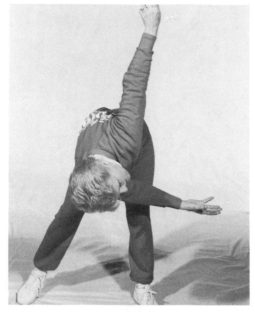

Leg Lifts to Back—Bend over at the waist, hands on a chair or solid surface. Lift the right leg and hold your head up at the same time. Arch the back. This is great for the hips, lower back and shoulders. Do this one 5 times on each leg.

Windmills—This is one of my favorites. Bend forward at the waist, arms stretched out. Simultaneously swing your right arm across your body and try to touch your left hand to the ceiling; then swing back your left arm and extend the right hand to the ceiling. Do this one rapidly, repeating it 10-20 times.

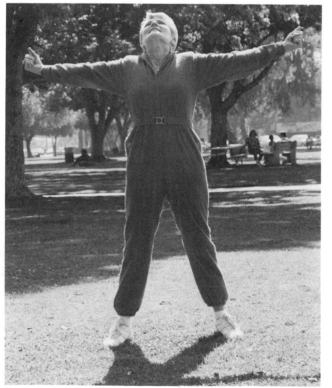

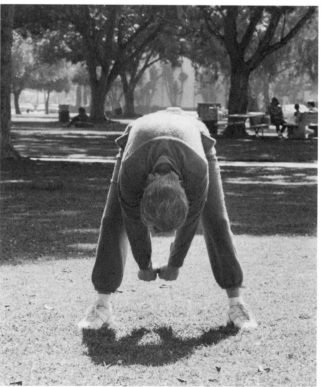

Dynamic Breath—Breathe in deeply through the nose, thrusting the arms out, looking up at the ceiling. Then, bend over at the waist and let the air out slowly through the mouth. Repeat 2-4 times. Ahhhhhh! That feels good!

58

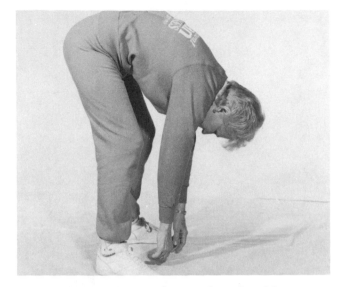

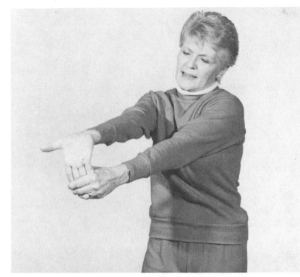

Rag Doll Stretch—With your feet shoulder-width apart, bend at the waist, legs straight; try to keep your back flat and allow your arms to hang loosely. Relax. Don't bounce. Allow gravity to do the work. Hold for a count of 10 and then shake all over. Repeat 5 times.

Hand Stretch—With the right arm and hand extended, use the left hand to pull the fingers back as far as possible. Don't go so far back you cause pain—just enough to stretch them. Repeat with the other hand. Hold for a count of 5 each time, and repeat 10 times on each side.

Special Top Secret Exercises

I'm a laugher. I love to laugh. My mother used to say, "Elaine was born laughing." I feel that a person who is happy, who has the capacity to laugh and see the humor in life, tends to be healthier. A friend of ours, Norman Cousins, has written a book about how laughter helped him through his cancer crisis. Researchers are continually proving that laughter is great medicine. There are researchers, too, who believe certain types of cancer and other diseases seem to gravitate toward people who are perpetually depressed and negative about life.

A good laugh is also good exercise. Although it takes more muscles to frown than it does to laugh, a laugh works a multitude of muscles throughout the body that a frown can't reach.

I have a couple of laughter-inducing exercises that I'd like to share with you. Recently I toured the country doing "Rut Buster" mall walks for people over 50 on behalf of Post Natural Bran Flakes. I included these in my warm-up sessions and each time I did, everyone seemed to get a laugh while doing them because they look so funny. They may look funny, but they benefit the legs, ankles and feet—the parts that do most of the work when we walk.

Do them in front of a full-length mirror and you'll see what I mean.

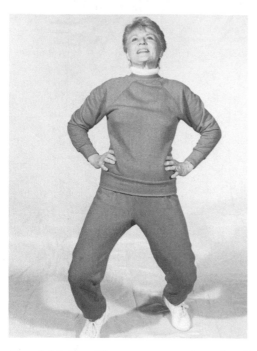

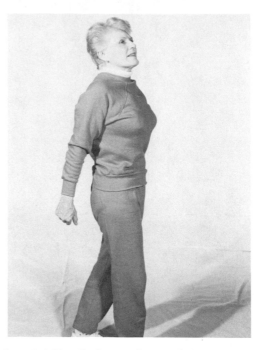

The Duck Walk—These are exercises that I do to get loosened up physically, and also to limber up my funny bone. They're funny and they're fun, and they utilize muscles that don't normally get enough attention. Standing with your feet shoulder-width apart, bend knees into a half-squat. Lean body slightly to back (like a lean-to). Now march forward and backward like a duck. Do this 3 or 4 times. Feel the thigh and abdominal muscles contracting.

Walnut Walk—Jack taught me this one many years ago. It's wonderful for the back and shoulders, hips and abdominal region. Pretend that you're holding a walnut between your shoulder blades, and try to crack it. At the same time, try to crack an imaginary walnut between your seat. Notice how your posture improves and your stomach muscles become nice and tight. In this position, walk around the room. Relax and repeat.

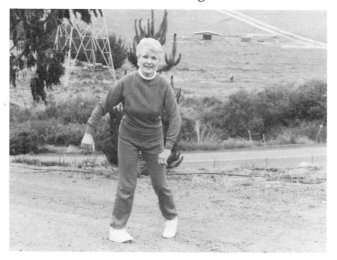

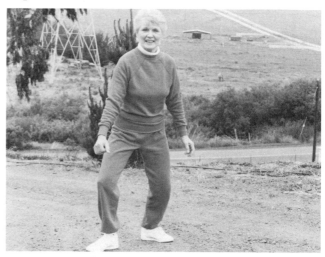

Pigeon-Toed Walk—This is another good one to work muscles you usually ignore. Point your toes inward and walk forward 20 steps, then walk backwards 20 more steps. Feel those legs stretch? Repeat this one 3 or 4 times in each direction. It works leg muscles that don't normally get worked when you walk.

Open-Toed Walk—Attempt to turn your feet outward. Now walk, very slowly, for 5 or 6 steps. Then walk backwards.

Exercises For Those "Slow-Out-Of-Bed" Days

Did you ever have one of those days when you really don't feel like getting out of bed even though you've got a thousand things to do?

I've got a series of warm-up exercises that I save as a warm-up to the real warm-up exercises for just those kinds of days.

All of these exercises are fairly easy and can be done in bed, as you'll see by looking at the pictures.

They *do* get your blood flowing and loosen up your body so by the time you're finished, you're energized enough to jump out of bed and, as my mother used to say, "Get going on the Get Going Program."

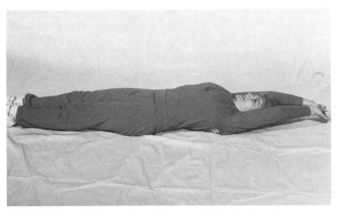

Wall-To-Wall Stretch—This and the following exercises are terrific for getting you up and out of bed. Lying on your back, point your toes toward the wall in front of you and stretch your hands as far as they'll go over your head, trying to touch the wall behind you. Make those muscles stretch as far as they'll go. Hold for a count of 5, relax, then repeat the exercise 5 times.

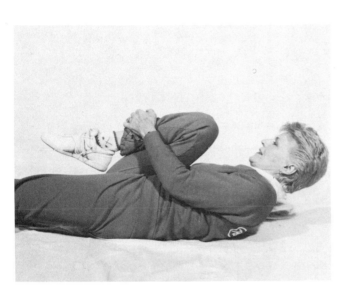

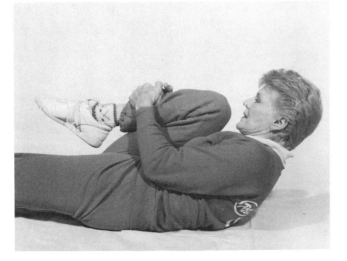

Knee-To-Chin Stretch—Lying on your back, grasp your right shin with both hands, then pull your knee toward your chin. Hold for a count of 5, and relax. Repeat 5 times on each leg.

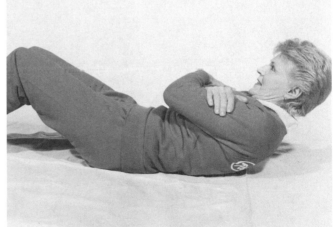

Crunches (Half Sit-Up)—Lying flat on your back, bend your knees, keeping your heels as close to your buttocks as possible, feet flat on the floor. Now, try to sit up to your knees. Exhale as you sit up; inhale as you lie down. Repeat 4 or 5 times at first, more as you become stronger.

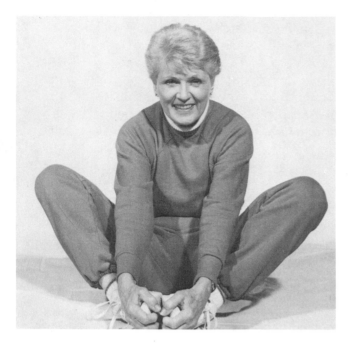

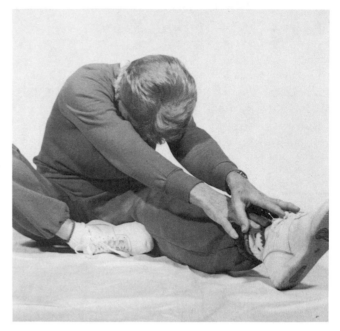

Inner Thigh Stretch—Sit up in bed and bring the soles of your feet together. Use your hands to hold them in position, and then gently attempt to touch your knees to the surface of the bed by lowering them. Don't push them into the pain zone. Hold for a count of 2, and return to the starting position. Repeat this one 5 times.

Toe-Touch Stretch—Sitting on the bed or floor, stretch your left leg out in front of you and bring the sole of your right foot flush against the inner segment of your left thigh. Now, bending at the waist, attempt to touch the toes of your left foot. Hold for a count of 2. Repeat 5 times on each leg.

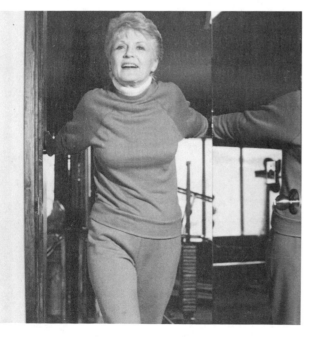

Doorway Stretch—Hold onto the framework on both sides of a door and then gently attempt to walk forward as far as you can, stretching your arms. Back up and repeat the process 5 times.

Chapter 7

Goals Within Reach

"It is good to collect things; it is better to walk."

—Anatole France

Suppose, for a moment, that you are visiting the Empire State Building in New York. You want to get to the top, but the elevators are out. How would you get there? You obviously can't jump or fly. After some consideration, you might conclude that you'd have to use the stairs.

Some people might run up the stairs, but by running they might very well give up halfway before they made it. Some might take two steps at a time. But even that can be tiring to the average person, and once again, may leave you far from the top. Other, more cautious people might take one step at a time until they reach the first floor. Then take one step at a time until they reach the second floor. Then on to the third . . . Until they finally reach their goal: the top of the building.

There's no doubt about it: to look up to the top of a building that seems impossible to reach under your own power seems overwhelming. And that's just the kind of overwhelmed feeling many of us get when we look up and see our long-range goals so far off, so distant.

By breaking down the long-range goal into a series of short-range goals, we are better able to handle the task of reaching them because they do not seem so overwhelming. Just like the person who took one step at a time until the first floor was reached, and then repeated the same process to the second, and so forth, until the top of the build-

ing was reached. What might have seemed like an impossible goal at first become achievable.

The analogy of the Empire State Building is similar to climbing to the roof of your house on a ladder, one rung at a time until you reach your roof. Your roof is your long-range goal and each rung corresponds to a short-term goal.

Have you ever noticed how, when we set outrageously high goals for ourselves, we frequently find it impossible to reach them?

The way I see it, there are two types of goals to consider: short-term and long-range.

I feel it is best to set reasonable goals, reach them and then set another reasonable goal and reach that. A long-range goal can more easily be reached by stringing together a series of short-term goals.

Avoid the two extremes. Don't set short-term goals that are so easy to reach that you never get off the ground. And don't set such difficult, far-away long-range goals that they are impossible to reach.

Make your goals reasonable and achievable. Your goals are your desires. No one else can make a goal *for you but you*.

I'd like to share one of my philosophies with you:

Yesterday has gone and tomorrow isn't here yet. You can't live in yesterday and you can't live in tomorrow. You can only live today. You can only live right now! Whether you realize it or not, what you look and feel like today is the culmination of the goals you set for yourself in the past; you are therefore living today the goals you set for yourself yesterday. If you are unhappy with the outcome of the old goals, you can set some new ones, because tomorrow has not yet come. Take one day at a time, one week at a time, one month at a time. Try to make every day count.

In other words, make your short-term goals fit your lifestyle and make them reachable in a reasonable amount of time. Don't frustrate yourself by making them too difficult. Short-term goals are the stepping stones to your long-range goals.

Long-range goals are extremely important because, as I said in my first book, *Fitness After 50*, without a long-range goal, we are like boats without rudders. We're going around in circles. Sometimes long-range goals seem so far away and unattainable that we tend to get sidetracked and instead of starting out again, we take the easy way out: we give up. Just because something comes along to disrupt the time frame you've set down for yourself, don't give up: take the pressure off yourself, forget the time frame, make a new one that is more realistic, but always keep in mind your ultimate goal.

When I was 19 my mother gave me a book called *Something to Live By* by Dorothea Kopplin. It was a book of quotations: everything from the Bible to Abraham Lincoln. There were a number of quotations from that book that have stuck in my mind, but one in particular is always foremost:

"Tis the set of the soul that decides the goal and not the storms of life."

Many storms do come into our lives to try to throw us off track, but if your desire is strong enough, that desire will weather any storm. Anything the mind can conceive it can achieve.

I think that because I was a cheerleader in high school, I feel like I want to send out a rousing cheer when I see people decide on a goal, take control of their lives by getting up on their feet and then do something for their health through fitness. I've been fortunate to travel throughout the country not only speaking about fitness, but leading groups of people, young and old, in warm-up exercises and participating in walking programs.

It is exhilarating to be among such vibrant, exciting individuals who have taken up this initiative. It is so very different from being among those of the same age who have given up the ghost before the ghost was ready to give up on them. To hear the personal testimonials of the walkers who are achieving amazing results from their programs stimulates me to try to motivate more and more individuals to a healthier life.

I remember meeting Anne. She was suffering from "flabby-seat-itis." She took up walking and watched what she put in her mouth. She remembered Jack's TV statement that what you eat today is walking and talking tomorrow. Voila! In a few months Anne dropped 20 pounds. At the same time, she firmed up her hips, thighs and waistline. Her friends all told her she looked 10 years younger. Now that was something to cheer about: a new body, a new image, and renewed self-esteem.

On another one of my walks with the seniors, I met a lady with determination that just could not be stopped. She had a pronounced limp from hip and knee problems, but that didn't slow her down. She finished eight out of 10 laps we attempted. She had to work harder than the other walkers to achieve her goals, but her doctors assured her that if she wanted to do it, the walking could do nothing but help her. Was she enthusiastic!

Many of the people I talk to at these walking events tell me that, in the past, they had become either bored with exercise, burned out by doing too much too soon, or had not been physically active since high school or college. However, when they took up a walking program, they approached it with a new attitude, new goals, renewed determination to stick to it, and with the knowledge you don't have to do it all overnight. Some were walking in malls, some in parks and others were walking at their health club so that they not only had the benefit of weight training equipment but also a walking and running track.

Those who had been on a program for more than three months were sold on walking for the rest of their lives. They could see the results: more energy reserves, more flexibility, weight loss, better muscle tone and a purpose in their day, around which they could focus other things.

On one of my walks I met a beautiful lady who told me she had taken up walking, cut down on what she put in her mouth and lost 67 pounds in seven months. She looked fantastic and said that she not only feels younger, but believe me, she looks younger.

Then there was Frank, 62, who started mall walking a year ago. His blood pressure has come from high to normal for his age, and he's managed to make plenty of new friends in the process.

My role as a walking cheerleader for these people is easy because they have found that a regularly-practiced, sensible walking program *does*

work and they end up being cheerleaders for themselves. When you are a good example to yourself, you can then encourage others to bring positive results into their lives, too: one step at a time.

It doesn't matter if you're a veteran of a dozen 26-mile marathon races or whether you have never exercised a day in your life.

Almost anyone can walk.

This is one fitness program in which you *can* succeed, and from which you can benefit in a variety of ways.

As we move into Part II of this book, remember the Three Commandments of Walking:

1. Set Realistic Goals.
2. Practice Regularity in Your Program.
3. Don't Attempt to Take on Too Much Too Soon.

PART II

Walking Is For You!

Chapter 8

The One-Day-At-A-Time Starter's Program

"Afoot and light-hearted I take to the open road."

"Song of the Open Road"
—Walt Whitman

There is a saying that even the longest trip begins with a single step.

That is the basis of this program. It begins with one simple step and progresses slowly and cautiously for the initial month of familiarization with a regular walking program. It essentially starts up your motor.

Who This Program Is For. This starter program is designed for those of you who have never exercised or for those who haven't exercised in quite some time.

Many of you may have been athletic at one point in your life, but did not keep at it. The benefits of athletics wear off very quickly if they are not maintained faithfully. In fact, if not used, a muscle starts to atrophy in a short time.

This program is also for those people whose medical test results caution them to begin with a conservative program. If in doubt, show this program to your family physician before embarking on the workouts. Remember this program is based not upon distance, but upon time and pulse rate (effort).

Those Who Can Skip This Program. This program is not designed for people who have remained at least relatively active and those who have no health restrictions as far as a regular exercise program is concerned. If you are already moderately fit, you can skip this chapter and proceed to Chapter 9.

"X" used in conjunction with a Free Day simply means that there are no readings and measurements taken for that day.

My Working Heart Rate
60% = _____ bpm
70% = _____ bpm
80% = _____ bpm

WEEK 1

	SUNDAY	MONDAY	TUESDAY
Resting Pulse Rate	_____ bpm	_____ bpm	_____ bpm
Warm-Up Exercises	( ) YES ( ) NO	( ) YES ( ) NO	( ) YES ( ) NO
Total Scheduled Walking Time	**10** minutes	**10** minutes	**FREE DAY**
Working Heart Rate	**60** % =____bpm	**60** % =____bpm	**X** % =____bpm
Type Course (Profile)	(X) Flat ( ) Hilly ( ) Mixed	(X) Flat ( ) Hilly ( ) Mixed	( ) Flat ( ) Hilly ( ) Mixed
Air Temperature	0	0	0
Walk Status: (Alone vs. with others)	( ) Alone ( ) With: _____	( ) Alone ( ) With: _____	( ) Alone ( ) With: _____
Cool-Down Exercises	( ) YES ( ) NO	( ) YES ( ) NO	( ) YES ( ) NO
Notes/Comments On Today's Walk			

bpm = beats per minute

WEDNESDAY	THURSDAY	FRIDAY	SATURDAY
_____bpm	_____bpm	_____bpm	_____bpm
( ) YES ( ) NO	( ) YES ( ) NO	( ) YES ( ) NO	( ) YES ( ) NO
10 minutes	**10** minutes	**10** minutes	**FREE DAY**
60% = ___bpm	**60**% = ___bpm	**60**% = ___bpm	**X**% = ___bpm
(X) Flat ( ) Hilly ( ) Mixed	(X) Flat ( ) Hilly ( ) Mixed	(X) Flat ( ) Hilly ( ) Mixed	( ) Flat ( ) Hilly ( ) Mixed
0	0	0	0
( ) Alone ( ) With: _____ _____	( ) Alone ( ) With: _____ _____	( ) Alone ( ) With: _____ _____	( ) Alone ( ) With: _____ _____
( ) YES ( ) NO	( ) YES ( ) NO	( ) YES ( ) NO	( ) YES ( ) NO

bpm = beats per minute

My Working Heart Rate
60% = _____ bpm
70% = _____ bpm
80% = _____ bpm

WEEK 2

	SUNDAY	MONDAY	TUESDAY
Resting Pulse Rate	_____ bpm	_____ bpm	_____ bpm
Warm-Up Exercises	( ) YES ( ) NO	( ) YES ( ) NO	( ) YES ( ) NO
Total Scheduled Walking Time	**12** minutes	**10** minutes	**FREE DAY**
Working Heart Rate	**60** % = ___ bpm	**60** % = ___ bpm	**X** % = ___ bpm
Type Course (Profile)	(X) Flat ( ) Hilly ( ) Mixed	(X) Flat ( ) Hilly ( ) Mixed	( ) Flat ( ) Hilly ( ) Mixed
Air Temperature	0	0	0
Walk Status: (Alone vs. with others)	( ) Alone ( ) With: _____ _____	( ) Alone ( ) With: _____ _____	( ) Alone ( ) With: _____ _____
Cool-Down Exercises	( ) YES ( ) NO	( ) YES ( ) NO	( ) YES ( ) NO
Notes/Comments On Today's Walk			

bpm = beats per minute

WEDNESDAY	THURSDAY	FRIDAY	SATURDAY
_____ bpm	_____ bpm	_____ bpm	_____ bpm
( ) YES ( ) NO	( ) YES ( ) NO	( ) YES ( ) NO	( ) YES ( ) NO
12 minutes	**10** minutes	**10** minutes	**FREE DAY**
60 % = ___bpm	**60** % = ___bpm	**60** % = ___bpm	**X** % = ___bpm
(X) Flat ( ) Hilly ( ) Mixed	(X) Flat ( ) Hilly ( ) Mixed	(X) Flat ( ) Hilly ( ) Mixed	( ) Flat ( ) Hilly ( ) Mixed
0	0	0	0
( ) Alone ( ) With: _____ _____	( ) Alone ( ) With: _____ _____	( ) Alone ( ) With: _____ _____	( ) Alone ( ) With: _____ _____
( ) YES ( ) NO	( ) YES ( ) NO	( ) YES ( ) NO	( ) YES ( ) NO

bpm = beats per minute

My Working Heart Rate
60% = ____ bpm
70% = ____ bpm
80% = ____ bpm

WEEK 3

	SUNDAY	MONDAY	TUESDAY
Resting Pulse Rate	_____bpm	_____ bpm	_____ bpm
Warm-Up Exercises	( ) YES ( ) NO	( ) YES ( ) NO	( ) YES ( ) NO
Total Scheduled Walking Time	**15** minutes	**10** minutes	**FREE DAY**
Working Heart Rate	**60**% = __ bpm	**60**% = __ bpm	**X** % = __ bpm
Type Course (Profile)	(X) Flat ( ) Hilly ( ) Mixed	(X) Flat ( ) Hilly ( ) Mixed	( ) Flat ( ) Hilly ( ) Mixed
Air Temperature	0	0	0
Walk Status: (Alone vs. with others)	( ) Alone ( ) With: _____ _____	( ) Alone ( ) With: _____ _____	( ) Alone ( ) With: _____ _____
Cool-Down Exercises	( ) YES ( ) NO	( ) YES ( ) NO	( ) YES ( ) NO
Notes/Comments On Today's Walk			

bpm = beats per minute

WEDNESDAY	THURSDAY	FRIDAY	SATURDAY
_____ bpm	_____ bpm	_____ bpm	_____bpm
( ) YES ( ) NO	( ) YES ( ) NO	( ) YES ( ) NO	( ) YES ( ) NO
15 minutes	**10** minutes	**12** minutes	**FREE DAY**
60 % = ___bpm	**60** % = ___bpm	**60** % = ___bpm	**X** % = ___bpm
(X) Flat ( ) Hilly ( ) Mixed	(X) Flat ( ) Hilly ( ) Mixed	(X) Flat ( ) Hilly ( ) Mixed	( ) Flat ( ) Hilly ( ) Mixed
0	0	0	0
( ) Alone ( ) With: _____ _____	( ) Alone ( ) With: _____ _____	( ) Alone ( ) With: _____ _____	( ) Alone ( ) With: _____ _____
( ) YES ( ) NO	( ) YES ( ) NO	( ) YES ( ) NO	( ) YES ( ) NO

bpm = beats per minute

My Working Heart Rate
60% = _____ bpm
70% = _____ bpm
80% = _____ bpm

WEEK 4

	SUNDAY	MONDAY	TUESDAY
Resting Pulse Rate	_____ bpm	_____ bpm	_____ bpm
Warm-Up Exercises	( ) YES ( ) NO	( ) YES ( ) NO	( ) YES ( ) NO
Total Scheduled Walking Time	**20** minutes	**12** minutes	**FREE DAY**
Working Heart Rate	**60** % = ___ bpm	**60** % = ___ bpm	**X** % = ___ bpm
Type Course (Profile)	(X) Flat ( ) Hilly ( ) Mixed	(X) Flat ( ) Hilly ( ) Mixed	( ) Flat ( ) Hilly ( ) Mixed
Air Temperature	0	0	0
Walk Status: (Alone vs. with others)	( ) Alone ( ) With:_____ _____	( ) Alone ( ) With:_____ _____	( ) Alone ( ) With:_____ _____
Cool-Down Exercises	( ) YES ( ) NO	( ) YES ( ) NO	( ) YES ( ) NO
Notes/Comments On Today's Walk			

bpm = beats per minute

WEDNESDAY	THURSDAY	FRIDAY	SATURDAY
_____bpm	_____bpm	_____bpm	_____bpm
( ) YES ( ) NO	( ) YES ( ) NO	( ) YES ( ) NO	( ) YES ( ) NO
20 minutes	**12** minutes	**15** minutes	**FREE DAY**
60 % = ___bpm	**60** % = ___bpm	**60** % = ___bpm	**X** % = ___bpm
(**X**) Flat ( ) Hilly ( ) Mixed	(**X**) Flat ( ) Hilly ( ) Mixed	(**X**) Flat ( ) Hilly ( ) Mixed	( ) Flat ( ) Hilly ( ) Mixed
0	0	0	0
( ) Alone ( ) With:_____ _____	( ) Alone ( ) With:_____ _____	( ) Alone ( ) With:_____ _____	( ) Alone ( ) With:_____ _____
( ) YES ( ) NO	( ) YES ( ) NO	( ) YES ( ) NO	( ) YES ( ) NO

bpm = beats per minute

Important Points to Remember

The following are presented to further explain the program:

1. If, at any time during the starter's program, you experience a shortness of breath or chest pains, please consult your physician immediately. Do *not* continue exercising until the cause of the discomfort has been determined.

2. Part of your warm-up and cool-down exercise is walking itself. If the starter's program for a specific day calls for 12 minutes of vigorous walking with a 60% Working Heart Rate (WHR), the 12 minutes begins once your heart rate reaches its 60% level. This may require you to begin walking slowly, gradually increasing your effort until your pulse rate rises to the necessary 60%. At the end of the 12 minutes, come down off your vigorous walking by slowing your walking pace until you are merely strolling. Then, proceed with your cool-down exercises.

3. If, for some reason, you are unable to get your walking in on a day as it is scheduled, take that day as a rest day. Do *not* add the time you missed to the next day's schedule, and do not simply move your entire schedule back a day. Continue to take your regularly scheduled rest days (Free Day). The object is to make your walking program a *regular* part of your day, your week, your life. If you begin to miss your scheduled walks twice a week, drop back and begin this program over until you find you can do them with regularity.

4. In the box labeled "Notes and Comments on Today's Walk," fill in anything that comes to mind. If nothing comes to mind, leave it blank. It is merely a space where you can record your impressions of the walk, what you saw on the walk, and/ or how you felt for later reference.

Chapter 9
The 90-Day Miracle

"Every walk is a sort of crusade."
—Henry David Thoreau

For those of you who have progressed from the One-Day-At-A-Time Starter's Program (Chapter 8) and those who bring a fair amount of fitness to a walking program, the 90-day program that follows is a blend of further building a base and some ambitious advances at a sensible pace. The program incorporates the principles of hard/easy training to the week, to the month, and to the three-month plan. You will also notice that the hard/easy principle is applied to the number of days a week you are asked to walk. Some weeks will feature five days, others six.

If you look at the 90-Day Miracle Program over the entire 90 days (actually, it's 91 days, or 13 weeks), you will notice that the hard/easy approach to training permeates the entire structure of the program. Exercise followed by rest is the only way to improve.

If you are happy with the level you reach at the end of the 13 weeks, return to Week 1 and repeat the schedule over and over again. By doing so, the hard/easy principles will repeat themselves, giving the athlete-walker four peaks and four restful valleys in each year.

For the more ambitious, there is always the next step, which is the subject of Chapter 10. If, for any reason you must interrupt your program, it may not be necessary to drop all the way back to the beginning. If the interruption is of no more than a week's duration, simply go back to your last full week, and then count back four weeks and restart at that point. Your body should readapt to the program.

If, however, the interruption exceeds one week, drop back to the beginning of the 90-day program, and start over. If the interruption is a month or more, evaluate how you feel physically, and then consider dropping back to redo Chapter 8 in order to re-establish a training base before proceeding with this more ambitious walking program.

My Working Heart Rate
60% = _____ bpm
70% = _____ bpm
80% = _____ bpm

WEEK 1

	SUNDAY	**MONDAY**	**TUESDAY**
Resting Pulse Rate	_____bpm	_____ bpm	_____ bpm
Warm-Up Exercises	( ) YES ( ) NO	( ) YES ( ) NO	( ) YES ( ) NO
Total Scheduled Walking Time	**20** minutes	**12** minutes	**FREE DAY**
Working Heart Rate	**60** % =____bpm	**60** % =____bpm	**X** % =____bpm
Type Course (Profile)	( ) Flat ( ) Hilly ( ) Mixed	( ) Flat ( ) Hilly ( ) Mixed	( ) Flat ( ) Hilly ( ) Mixed
Air Temperature	0	0	0
Walk Status: (Alone vs. with others)	( ) Alone ( ) With: _____ _____	( ) Alone ( ) With: _____ _____	( ) Alone ( ) With: _____ _____
Cool-Down Exercises	( ) YES ( ) NO	( ) YES ( ) NO	( ) YES ( ) NO
Notes/Comments On Today's Walk			

bpm = beats per minute

WEDNESDAY	THURSDAY	FRIDAY	SATURDAY
_____bpm	_____bpm	_____bpm	_____bpm
( ) YES ( ) NO	( ) YES ( ) NO	( ) YES ( ) NO	( ) YES ( ) NO
20 minutes	**12** minutes	**15** minutes	**FREE DAY**
70 % = ___bpm	**60** % = ___bpm	**70** % = ___bpm	**X** % = ___bpm
( ) Flat ( ) Hilly ( ) Mixed	( ) Flat ( ) Hilly ( ) Mixed	( ) Flat ( ) Hilly ( ) Mixed	( ) Flat ( ) Hilly ( ) Mixed
0	0	0	0
( ) Alone ( ) With:_____ _____	( ) Alone ( ) With:_____ _____	( ) Alone ( ) With:_____ _____	( ) Alone ( ) With:_____ _____
( ) YES ( ) NO	( ) YES ( ) NO	( ) YES ( ) NO	( ) YES ( ) NO

bpm = beats per minute

My Working Heart Rate
60% = ____ bpm
70% = ____ bpm
80% = ____ bpm

WEEK 2

	SUNDAY	MONDAY	TUESDAY
Resting Pulse Rate	_____bpm	_____bpm	_____bpm
Warm-Up Exercises	( ) YES ( ) NO	( ) YES ( ) NO	( ) YES ( ) NO
Total Scheduled Walking Time	**20** minutes	**15** minutes	**FREE DAY**
Working Heart Rate	**70**% = ___bpm	**60**% = ___bpm	**X**% = ___bpm
Type Course (Profile)	( ) Flat ( ) Hilly ( ) Mixed	( ) Flat ( ) Hilly ( ) Mixed	( ) Flat ( ) Hilly ( ) Mixed
Air Temperature	0	0	0
Walk Status: (Alone vs. with others)	( ) Alone ( ) With:_____	( ) Alone ( ) With:_____	( ) Alone ( ) With:_____
Cool-Down Exercises	( ) YES ( ) NO	( ) YES ( ) NO	( ) YES ( ) NO
Notes/Comments On Today's Walk			

bpm = beats per minute

WEDNESDAY	THURSDAY	FRIDAY	SATURDAY
_____bpm	_____bpm	_____bpm	_____bpm
( ) YES ( ) NO	( ) YES ( ) NO	( ) YES ( ) NO	( ) YES ( ) NO
20 minutes	**12** minutes	**20** minutes	**15** minutes
70 % = ___bpm	**60** % = ___bpm	**60** % = ___bpm	**60** % = ___bpm
( ) Flat ( ) Hilly ( ) Mixed	( ) Flat ( ) Hilly ( ) Mixed	( ) Flat ( ) Hilly ( ) Mixed	( ) Flat ( ) Hilly ( ) Mixed
0	0	0	0
( ) Alone ( ) With:_____ _____	( ) Alone ( ) With:_____ _____	( ) Alone ( ) With:_____ _____	( ) Alone ( ) With:_____ _____
( ) YES ( ) NO	( ) YES ( ) NO	( ) YES ( ) NO	( ) YES ( ) NO

bpm = beats per minute

My Working Heart Rate
60% = _____ bpm
70% = _____ bpm
80% = _____ bpm

WEEK 3

	SUNDAY	MONDAY	TUESDAY
Resting Pulse Rate	_____ bpm	_____ bpm	_____ bpm
Warm-Up Exercises	( ) YES ( ) NO	( ) YES ( ) NO	( ) YES ( ) NO
Total Scheduled Walking Time	**20** minutes	**15** minutes	**FREE DAY**
Working Heart Rate	**70**% = ___bpm	**60**% = ___bpm	**X**% = ___bpm
Type Course (Profile)	( ) Flat ( ) Hilly ( ) Mixed	( ) Flat ( ) Hilly ( ) Mixed	( ) Flat ( ) Hilly ( ) Mixed
Air Temperature	0	0	0
Walk Status: (Alone vs. with others)	( ) Alone ( ) With: _____ _____	( ) Alone ( ) With: _____ _____	( ) Alone ( ) With: _____ _____
Cool-Down Exercises	( ) YES ( ) NO	( ) YES ( ) NO	( ) YES ( ) NO
Notes/Comments On Today's Walk			

bpm = beats per minute

WEDNESDAY	THURSDAY	FRIDAY	SATURDAY
_____bpm	_____bpm	_____bpm	_____bpm
( ) YES ( ) NO	( ) YES ( ) NO	( ) YES ( ) NO	( ) YES ( ) NO
25 minutes	**15** minutes	**20** minutes	**FREE DAY**
60 % = ___bpm	**60** % = ___bpm	**60** % = ___bpm	**X** % = ___bpm
( ) Flat ( ) Hilly ( ) Mixed	( ) Flat ( ) Hilly ( ) Mixed	( ) Flat ( ) Hilly ( ) Mixed	( ) Flat ( ) Hilly ( ) Mixed
0	0	0	0
( ) Alone ( ) With:_____ _____	( ) Alone ( ) With:_____ _____	( ) Alone ( ) With:_____ _____	( ) Alone ( ) With:_____ _____
( ) YES ( ) NO	( ) YES ( ) NO	( ) YES ( ) NO	( ) YES ( ) NO

bpm = beats per minute

My Working Heart Rate
60% = ____ bpm
70% = ____ bpm
80% = ____ bpm

WEEK 4

	SUNDAY	MONDAY	TUESDAY
Resting Pulse Rate	_____bpm	_____bpm	_____bpm
Warm-Up Exercises	( ) YES ( ) NO	( ) YES ( ) NO	( ) YES ( ) NO
Total Scheduled Walking Time	**25** minutes	**15** minutes	**FREE DAY**
Working Heart Rate	**60** % = ___bpm	**60** % = ___bpm	**X** % = ___bpm
Type Course (Profile)	( ) Flat ( ) Hilly ( ) Mixed	( ) Flat ( ) Hilly ( ) Mixed	( ) Flat ( ) Hilly ( ) Mixed
Air Temperature	0	0	0
Walk Status: (Alone vs. with others)	( ) Alone ( ) With:_____ _____	( ) Alone ( ) With:_____ _____	( ) Alone ( ) With:_____ _____
Cool-Down Exercises	( ) YES ( ) NO	( ) YES ( ) NO	( ) YES ( ) NO
Notes/Comments On Today's Walk			

bpm = beats per minute

WEDNESDAY	THURSDAY	FRIDAY	SATURDAY
_____bpm	_____bpm	_____bpm	_____bpm
( ) YES ( ) NO	( ) YES ( ) NO	( ) YES ( ) NO	( ) YES ( ) NO
25 minutes	**15** minutes	**20** minutes	**15** minutes
70 % = ___bpm	**60** % = ___bpm	**60** % = ___bpm	**60** % = ___bpm
( ) Flat ( ) Hilly ( ) Mixed	( ) Flat ( ) Hilly ( ) Mixed	( ) Flat ( ) Hilly ( ) Mixed	( ) Flat ( ) Hilly ( ) Mixed
0	0	0	0
( ) Alone ( ) With:_____ _____	( ) Alone ( ) With:_____ _____	( ) Alone ( ) With:_____ _____	( ) Alone ( ) With:_____ _____
( ) YES ( ) NO	( ) YES ( ) NO	( ) YES ( ) NO	( ) YES ( ) NO

bpm = beats per minute

My Working Heart Rate
60% = _____ bpm
70% = _____ bpm
80% = _____ bpm

WEEK 5

	SUNDAY	**MONDAY**	**TUESDAY**
Resting Pulse Rate	_____bpm	_____bpm	_____bpm
Warm-Up Exercises	( ) YES ( ) NO	( ) YES ( ) NO	( ) YES ( ) NO
Total Scheduled Walking Time	**20** minutes	**15** minutes	**FREE DAY**
Working Heart Rate	**70**% =____bpm	**60**% =____bpm	**X**% =____bpm
Type Course (Profile)	( ) Flat ( ) Hilly ( ) Mixed	( ) Flat ( ) Hilly ( ) Mixed	( ) Flat ( ) Hilly ( ) Mixed
Air Temperature	0	0	0
Walk Status: (Alone vs. with others)	( ) Alone ( ) With:_____ _____	( ) Alone ( ) With:_____ _____	( ) Alone ( ) With:_____ _____
Cool-Down Exercises	( ) YES ( ) NO	( ) YES ( ) NO	( ) YES ( ) NO
Notes/Comments On Today's Walk			

bpm = beats per minute

WEDNESDAY	THURSDAY	FRIDAY	SATURDAY
_____bpm	_____bpm	_____bpm	_____bpm
( ) YES ( ) NO	( ) YES ( ) NO	( ) YES ( ) NO	( ) YES ( ) NO
20 minutes	**12** minutes	**20** minutes	**FREE DAY**
70 % = ___bpm	**60** % = ___bpm	**60** % = ___bpm	**X** % = ___bpm
( ) Flat ( ) Hilly ( ) Mixed	( ) Flat ( ) Hilly ( ) Mixed	( ) Flat ( ) Hilly ( ) Mixed	( ) Flat ( ) Hilly ( ) Mixed
0	0	0	0
( ) Alone ( ) With:_____ _____	( ) Alone ( ) With:_____ _____	( ) Alone ( ) With:_____ _____	( ) Alone ( ) With:_____ _____
( ) YES ( ) NO	( ) YES ( ) NO	( ) YES ( ) NO	( ) YES ( ) NO

bpm = beats per minute

My Working Heart Rate
60% = ____ bpm
70% = ____ bpm
80% = ____ bpm

WEEK   6

	SUNDAY	**MONDAY**	**TUESDAY**
Resting Pulse Rate	_____ bpm	_____ bpm	_____ bpm
Warm-Up Exercises	( ) YES ( ) NO	( ) YES ( ) NO	( ) YES ( ) NO
Total Scheduled Walking Time	**25** minutes	**15** minutes	**FREE DAY**
Working Heart Rate	**60** % = ___ bpm	**60** % = ___ bpm	**X** % = ___ bpm
Type Course (Profile)	( ) Flat ( ) Hilly ( ) Mixed	( ) Flat ( ) Hilly ( ) Mixed	( ) Flat ( ) Hilly ( ) Mixed
Air Temperature	0	0	0
Walk Status: (Alone vs. with others)	( ) Alone ( ) With: _____ _____	( ) Alone ( ) With: _____ _____	( ) Alone ( ) With: _____ _____
Cool-Down Exercises	( ) YES ( ) NO	( ) YES ( ) NO	( ) YES ( ) NO
Notes/Comments On Today's Walk			

bpm = beats per minute

WEDNESDAY	THURSDAY	FRIDAY	SATURDAY
_____bpm	_____bpm	_____bpm	_____bpm
( ) YES ( ) NO	( ) YES ( ) NO	( ) YES ( ) NO	( ) YES ( ) NO
25 minutes	**15** minutes	**20** minutes	**20** minutes
70% = ___bpm	**60**% = ___bpm	**70**% = ___bpm	**60**% = ___bpm
( ) Flat ( ) Hilly ( ) Mixed	( ) Flat ( ) Hilly ( ) Mixed	( ) Flat ( ) Hilly ( ) Mixed	( ) Flat ( ) Hilly ( ) Mixed
0	0	0	0
( ) Alone ( ) With:_____ _____	( ) Alone ( ) With:_____ _____	( ) Alone ( ) With:_____ _____	( ) Alone ( ) With:_____ _____
( ) YES ( ) NO	( ) YES ( ) NO	( ) YES ( ) NO	( ) YES ( ) NO

bpm = beats per minute

My Working Heart Rate
60% = ____ bpm
70% = ____ bpm
80% = ____ bpm

WEEK 7

	SUNDAY	MONDAY	TUESDAY
Resting Pulse Rate	_____ bpm	_____ bpm	_____ bpm
Warm-Up Exercises	( ) YES ( ) NO	( ) YES ( ) NO	( ) YES ( ) NO
Total Scheduled Walking Time	**30** minutes	**20** minutes	**FREE DAY**
Working Heart Rate	60 % = ___bpm	60 % = ___bpm	X % = ___bpm
Type Course (Profile)	( ) Flat ( ) Hilly ( ) Mixed	( ) Flat ( ) Hilly ( ) Mixed	( ) Flat ( ) Hilly ( ) Mixed
Air Temperature	0	0	0
Walk Status: (Alone vs. with others)	( ) Alone ( ) With:_____ _____	( ) Alone ( ) With:_____ _____	( ) Alone ( ) With:_____ _____
Cool-Down Exercises	( ) YES ( ) NO	( ) YES ( ) NO	( ) YES ( ) NO
Notes/Comments On Today's Walk			

bpm = beats per minute

WEDNESDAY	THURSDAY	FRIDAY	SATURDAY
_____bpm	_____bpm	_____bpm	_____bpm
( ) YES ( ) NO	( ) YES ( ) NO	( ) YES ( ) NO	( ) YES ( ) NO
25 minutes	**20** minutes	**20** minutes	**FREE DAY**
70 % = ___bpm	**60** % = ___bpm	**60** % = ___bpm	**X** % = ___bpm
( ) Flat ( ) Hilly ( ) Mixed	( ) Flat ( ) Hilly ( ) Mixed	( ) Flat ( ) Hilly ( ) Mixed	( ) Flat ( ) Hilly ( ) Mixed
0	0	0	0
( ) Alone ( ) With:_____ _____	( ) Alone ( ) With:_____ _____	( ) Alone ( ) With:_____ _____	( ) Alone ( ) With:_____ _____
( ) YES ( ) NO	( ) YES ( ) NO	( ) YES ( ) NO	( ) YES ( ) NO

bpm = beats per minute

My Working Heart Rate
60% = _____ bpm
70% = _____ bpm
80% = _____ bpm

WEEK 8

	SUNDAY	MONDAY	TUESDAY
Resting Pulse Rate	_____ bpm	_____ bpm	_____ bpm
Warm-Up Exercises	( ) YES ( ) NO	( ) YES ( ) NO	( ) YES ( ) NO
Total Scheduled Walking Time	**30** minutes	**20** minutes	**FREE DAY**
Working Heart Rate	**70** % = ___bpm	**60** % = ___bpm	**X** % = ___bpm
Type Course (Profile)	( ) Flat ( ) Hilly ( ) Mixed	( ) Flat ( ) Hilly ( ) Mixed	( ) Flat ( ) Hilly ( ) Mixed
Air Temperature	0	0	0
Walk Status: (Alone vs. with others)	( ) Alone ( ) With: _____ _____	( ) Alone ( ) With: _____ _____	( ) Alone ( ) With: _____ _____
Cool-Down Exercises	( ) YES ( ) NO	( ) YES ( ) NO	( ) YES ( ) NO
Notes/Comments On Today's Walk			

bpm = beats per minute

WEDNESDAY	THURSDAY	FRIDAY	SATURDAY
_____bpm	_____bpm	_____bpm	_____bpm
( ) YES ( ) NO	( ) YES ( ) NO	( ) YES ( ) NO	( ) YES ( ) NO
30 minutes	**20** minutes	**25** minutes	**15** minutes
70 % = ___bpm	**60** % = ___bpm	**60** % = ___bpm	**60** % = ___bpm
( ) Flat ( ) Hilly ( ) Mixed	( ) Flat ( ) Hilly ( ) Mixed	( ) Flat ( ) Hilly ( ) Mixed	( ) Flat ( ) Hilly ( ) Mixed
0	0	0	0
( ) Alone ( ) With:_____ _____	( ) Alone ( ) With:_____ _____	( ) Alone ( ) With:_____ _____	( ) Alone ( ) With:_____ _____
( ) YES ( ) NO	( ) YES ( ) NO	( ) YES ( ) NO	( ) YES ( ) NO

bpm = beats per minute

My Working Heart Rate
60% = ___ bpm
70% = ___ bpm
80% = ___ bpm

WEEK 9

	SUNDAY	MONDAY	TUESDAY
Resting Pulse Rate	_____bpm	_____bpm	_____bpm
Warm-Up Exercises	( ) YES ( ) NO	( ) YES ( ) NO	( ) YES ( ) NO
Total Scheduled Walking Time	**25** minutes	**20** minutes	**FREE DAY**
Working Heart Rate	**60** % = ___bpm	**70** % = ___bpm	**X** % = ___bpm
Type Course (Profile)	( ) Flat ( ) Hilly ( ) Mixed	( ) Flat ( ) Hilly ( ) Mixed	( ) Flat ( ) Hilly ( ) Mixed
Air Temperature	0	0	0
Walk Status: (Alone vs. with others)	( ) Alone ( ) With:_____ _____	( ) Alone ( ) With:_____ _____	( ) Alone ( ) With:_____ _____
Cool-Down Exercises	( ) YES ( ) NO	( ) YES ( ) NO	( ) YES ( ) NO
Notes/Comments On Today's Walk			

bpm = beats per minute

WEDNESDAY	THURSDAY	FRIDAY	SATURDAY
_____bpm	_____bpm	_____bpm	_____bpm
( ) YES ( ) NO	( ) YES ( ) NO	( ) YES ( ) NO	( ) YES ( ) NO
30 minutes	**20** minutes	**30** minutes	**FREE DAY**
70 % = ___bpm	**60** % = ___bpm	**60** % = ___bpm	**X** % = ___bpm
( ) Flat ( ) Hilly ( ) Mixed	( ) Flat ( ) Hilly ( ) Mixed	( ) Flat ( ) Hilly ( ) Mixed	( ) Flat ( ) Hilly ( ) Mixed
0	0	0	0
( ) Alone ( ) With:_____ _____	( ) Alone ( ) With:_____ _____	( ) Alone ( ) With:_____ _____	( ) Alone ( ) With:_____ _____
( ) YES ( ) NO	( ) YES ( ) NO	( ) YES ( ) NO	( ) YES ( ) NO

bpm = beats per minute

My Working Heart Rate
60% = ____ bpm
70% = ____ bpm
80% = ____ bpm

WEEK 10

	SUNDAY	MONDAY	TUESDAY
Resting Pulse Rate	_____ bpm	_____ bpm	_____ bpm
Warm-Up Exercises	( ) YES ( ) NO	( ) YES ( ) NO	( ) YES ( ) NO
Total Scheduled Walking Time	**30** minutes	**25** minutes	**FREE DAY**
Working Heart Rate	**70** % = __bpm	**60** % = __bpm	**X** % = __bpm
Type Course (Profile)	( ) Flat ( ) Hilly ( ) Mixed	( ) Flat ( ) Hilly ( ) Mixed	( ) Flat ( ) Hilly ( ) Mixed
Air Temperature	0	0	0
Walk Status: (Alone vs. with others)	( ) Alone ( ) With: _____ _____	( ) Alone ( ) With: _____ _____	( ) Alone ( ) With: _____ _____
Cool-Down Exercises	( ) YES ( ) NO	( ) YES ( ) NO	( ) YES ( ) NO
Notes/Comments On Today's Walk			

bpm = beats per minute

WEDNESDAY	THURSDAY	FRIDAY	SATURDAY
_____bpm	_____bpm	_____bpm	_____bpm
( ) YES ( ) NO	( ) YES ( ) NO	( ) YES ( ) NO	( ) YES ( ) NO
35 minutes	**25** minutes	**30** minutes	**20** minutes
70 % = ___bpm	**60** % = ___bpm	**60** % = ___bpm	**60** % = ___bpm
( ) Flat ( ) Hilly ( ) Mixed	( ) Flat ( ) Hilly ( ) Mixed	( ) Flat ( ) Hilly ( ) Mixed	( ) Flat ( ) Hilly ( ) Mixed
0	0	0	0
( ) Alone ( ) With:_____ _____	( ) Alone ( ) With:_____ _____	( ) Alone ( ) With:_____ _____	( ) Alone ( ) With:_____ _____
( ) YES ( ) NO	( ) YES ( ) NO	( ) YES ( ) NO	( ) YES ( ) NO

bpm = beats per minute

My Working Heart Rate
60% = _____ bpm
70% = _____ bpm
80% = _____ bpm

WEEK 11

	SUNDAY	MONDAY	TUESDAY
Resting Pulse Rate	_____ bpm	_____ bpm	_____ bpm
Warm-Up Exercises	( ) YES ( ) NO	( ) YES ( ) NO	( ) YES ( ) NO
Total Scheduled Walking Time	**35** minutes	**30** minutes	**FREE DAY**
Working Heart Rate	**70** % = ___ bpm	**60** % = ___ bpm	**X** % = ___ bpm
Type Course (Profile)	( ) Flat ( ) Hilly ( ) Mixed	( ) Flat ( ) Hilly ( ) Mixed	( ) Flat ( ) Hilly ( ) Mixed
Air Temperature	0	0	0
Walk Status: (Alone vs. with others)	( ) Alone ( ) With:_____	( ) Alone ( ) With:_____	( ) Alone ( ) With:_____
Cool-Down Exercises	( ) YES ( ) NO	( ) YES ( ) NO	( ) YES ( ) NO
Notes/Comments On Today's Walk			

bpm = beats per minute

WEDNESDAY	THURSDAY	FRIDAY	SATURDAY
_____bpm	_____bpm	_____bpm	_____bpm
( ) YES ( ) NO	( ) YES ( ) NO	( ) YES ( ) NO	( ) YES ( ) NO
40 minutes	**30** minutes	**25** minutes	**FREE DAY**
70 % = ___bpm	**60** % = ___bpm	**70** % = ___bpm	**X** % = ___bpm
( ) Flat ( ) Hilly ( ) Mixed	( ) Flat ( ) Hilly ( ) Mixed	( ) Flat ( ) Hilly ( ) Mixed	( ) Flat ( ) Hilly ( ) Mixed
0	0	0	0
( ) Alone ( ) With:_____ _____	( ) Alone ( ) With:_____ _____	( ) Alone ( ) With:_____ _____	( ) Alone ( ) With:_____ _____
( ) YES ( ) NO	( ) YES ( ) NO	( ) YES ( ) NO	( ) YES ( ) NO

bpm = beats per minute

My Working Heart Rate
60% = _____ bpm
70% = _____ bpm
80% = _____ bpm

WEEK 12

	SUNDAY	MONDAY	TUESDAY
Resting Pulse Rate	_____ bpm	_____ bpm	_____ bpm
Warm-Up Exercises	( ) YES ( ) NO	( ) YES ( ) NO	( ) YES ( ) NO
Total Scheduled Walking Time	**40** minutes	**30** minutes	**FREE DAY**
Working Heart Rate	**70**% = ___bpm	**60** % = ___bpm	**X** % = ___bpm
Type Course (Profile)	( ) Flat ( ) Hilly ( ) Mixed	( ) Flat ( ) Hilly ( ) Mixed	( ) Flat ( ) Hilly ( ) Mixed
Air Temperature	0	0	0
Walk Status: (Alone vs. with others)	( ) Alone ( ) With: _____ _____	( ) Alone ( ) With: _____ _____	( ) Alone ( ) With: _____ _____
Cool-Down Exercises	( ) YES ( ) NO	( ) YES ( ) NO	( ) YES ( ) NO
Notes/Comments On Today's Walk			

bpm = beats per minute

WEDNESDAY	THURSDAY	FRIDAY	SATURDAY
_____bpm	_____bpm	_____bpm	_____bpm
( ) YES ( ) NO	( ) YES ( ) NO	( ) YES ( ) NO	( ) YES ( ) NO
40 minutes	**30** minutes	**30** minutes	**30** minutes
70 % = ___bpm	**60** % = ___bpm	**70** % = ___bpm	**60** % = ___bpm
( ) Flat ( ) Hilly ( ) Mixed	( ) Flat ( ) Hilly ( ) Mixed	( ) Flat ( ) Hilly ( ) Mixed	( ) Flat ( ) Hilly ( ) Mixed
0	0	0	0
( ) Alone ( ) With:_____ _____	( ) Alone ( ) With:_____ _____	( ) Alone ( ) With:_____ _____	( ) Alone ( ) With:_____ _____
( ) YES ( ) NO	( ) YES ( ) NO	( ) YES ( ) NO	( ) YES ( ) NO

bpm = beats per minute

My Working Heart Rate
60% = ____ bpm
70% = ____ bpm
80% = ____ bpm

WEEK 13

	SUNDAY	MONDAY	TUESDAY
Resting Pulse Rate	_____ bpm	_____ bpm	_____ bpm
Warm-Up Exercises	( ) YES ( ) NO	( ) YES ( ) NO	( ) YES ( ) NO
Total Scheduled Walking Time	**30** minutes	**20** minutes	**FREE DAY**
Working Heart Rate	**70**% = __bpm	**60**% = __bpm	**X**% = __bpm
Type Course (Profile)	( ) Flat ( ) Hilly ( ) Mixed	( ) Flat ( ) Hilly ( ) Mixed	( ) Flat ( ) Hilly ( ) Mixed
Air Temperature	0	0	0
Walk Status: (Alone vs. with others)	( ) Alone ( ) With: _____ _____	( ) Alone ( ) With: _____ _____	( ) Alone ( ) With: _____ _____
Cool-Down Exercises	( ) YES ( ) NO	( ) YES ( ) NO	( ) YES ( ) NO
Notes/Comments On Today's Walk			

bpm = beats per minute

WEDNESDAY	THURSDAY	FRIDAY	SATURDAY
_____bpm	_____bpm	_____bpm	_____bpm
( ) YES ( ) NO	( ) YES ( ) NO	( ) YES ( ) NO	( ) YES ( ) NO
30 minutes	**30** minutes	**30** minutes	**FREE DAY**
70 % = ___bpm	**60** % = ___bpm	**70** % = ___bpm	**X** % = ___bpm
( ) Flat ( ) Hilly ( ) Mixed	( ) Flat ( ) Hilly ( ) Mixed	( ) Flat ( ) Hilly ( ) Mixed	( ) Flat ( ) Hilly ( ) Mixed
0	0	0	0
( ) Alone ( ) With:_____ _____	( ) Alone ( ) With:_____ _____	( ) Alone ( ) With:_____ _____	( ) Alone ( ) With:_____ _____
( ) YES ( ) NO	( ) YES ( ) NO	( ) YES ( ) NO	( ) YES ( ) NO

When completed, either return to week 1 or move to Chapter 10

Important Points to Remember

1. It is not really necessary to vary courses for the starter's program (Chapter 8) due to the brevity of the workouts and the program. However, once you move into a program of more than a month, try mixing courses (as outlined in Chapter 4) in order to keep the program fresh and to stave off boredom. Some new exercisers will find absolutely no boredom in doing the same course day after day, year after year, because they find tremendous freedom and release in their workout; boredom is the last thing from their minds.

While taking pictures for the cover of this book, Jack an I met a young senior named Florence. Florence was walking with her friend Sarah, whom she'd met during a walk in the park. She declined to tell us her age, but with a twinkle in her eye and a smile on her face, said, "I'm the world's oldest lady." I said, "I doubt that." But she certainly had the world's youngest attitude. She had been walking in this same park for about four years. Her walking program was anything but boring to her.

For others, however, avoiding boredom is essential to continuing a program. So try to make variety a part of your program from the very start. Mix up your courses, using a different one every day of the week if you so desire. You may want to set up your courses so that you do similar workouts on the same course on similar days (Sunday, for instance) as a means of measuring your progress. After four weeks on the Chapter 9 program, do you walk farther in 20 minutes on your Sunday course than you did at the start of the program? That's *measurable* progress.

2. Some people, contemplating a 90-day program, would tend to think, "Good gracious! Ninety days! That'll take forever!" In actuality, 90 days goes by very, very quickly—if you make your walking program an integral part of your day! At the end of the 91 days, you'll say to yourself, "Where did all those days go? They were gone in absolutely no time at all!"

3. If at any time during the program you are unable to complete a week's workout, whether because of health problems or because of scheduling difficulties, drop back to the last comfortably completed week you had on the schedule (this is where your notes at the bottom of each day will come in handy), repeat that week, and then continue on with the program.

4. If you have even the hint of a leg, ankle or foot problem, have it checked immediately. Treat it or have it treated, and then continue cautiously until the problem is resolved to your satisfaction. Do *not* push yourself through pains in the legs, ankles or feet. Stop and take care of the problem. And then proceed with caution. It is your legs, ankles and feet that will carry you through these programs and on to fitness and health, so give them the best care you can.

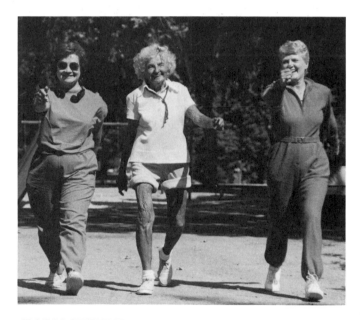

DYNASTRIDE, Everyone—Anyone can Dynastride almost anywhere they want. During our cover shoot, we met two dedicated walkers. Florence calls herself "the world's oldest lady," although she's anything but old as far as I'm concerned. Her walking buddy is Sarah. They met while walking their separate courses in the park. Now they walk together and are fast friends. Jack and I enjoyed visiting with them, even if our visit was in motion at all times. They were very interested in the additional benefits provided by Dynastriding.

Chapter 10

The Top-Of-The-Pyramid

"Unhappy businessmen, I am convinced, would increase their happiness more by walking six miles every day than by any conceivable change of philosophy."

—Bertrand Russell

Most people who take up an aerobic sport do so with one thing in mind: to get fit, and by getting fit, to improve their health or to guard against possible health risks (usually heart disease).

At least that's how people start out on their fitness programs.

Somewhere along the way, however, a certain number of these people—often the ones you would least expect—get it into their mind that they want to do more than just become fit because they see the good results of their training. These results often lure them further onward to taste more of the benefits.

Therefore, the following one-year program is for those who want to get even more results, and who have proven, to a doctor's satisfaction, that after successfully completing Chapter 9, you are capable of physically making a more ambitious commitment. (For those who are quite content with the improvements that have come with the walking program just completed, either repeat the program every time you reach the end, or move on to Chapter 11.)

The Top-Of-The-Pyramid Program covers a full year. Not only can you take advantage of the benefits of the hard/easy theory of training, but it is designed to raise your fitness level significantly at the 9-10 month point.

There is no set time of the year when the program must be started. But when you do start, pay close attention to your body's adaptation to this program. If you encounter problems, *do not* go beyond your capacity. Either consult your doctor to determine the problem, or drop back a full four weeks in the program and restart from there. It may be that you have found your natural peak capacity for exercise at this point. It is *always* better to be on the side of too little than on the side of doing too much.

You'll notice that there are some suggested variations thrown into this program at strategic points. If you ride a bike, try bicycle riding instead of a rest day here and there, walking hills instead of walking on the level, and an occasional very long walk to further build endurance and strength, or just take the day off to rest.

As you engage in this program, I would advise you to consult with your physician on a regular basis; he is able to give you medical input as well as monitor your blood pressure, resting pulse rate, and other indicators with more sophisticated equipment than you might normally use.

My Working Heart Rate
60% = _____ bpm
70% = _____ bpm
80% = _____ bpm

WEEKS 1 — 4

WEEK 1

	SUN	MON	TUE	WED	THU	FRI	SAT
Resting Pulse Rate							
Walking Time	25	20	Free	25	30	25	25
W. H. R.	70	60	X	70	60	70	60
Course Profile	F	F	X	F	F	F	F
Air Temperature			X				
Notes/Comments							

WEEK 2

	SUN	MON	TUE	WED	THU	FRI	SAT
Resting Pulse Rate							
Walking Time	30	20	Free	30	30	30	Bike
W.H. R.	70	60	X	70	60	70	X
Course Profile	F	F	X	M	F	F	X
Air Temperature			X				
Notes/Comments							

Under "Course Profile": F = Flat, H = Hilly, M = Mixed

REMEMBER: When the schedule calls for a Free Day, either take the day off from exercise walking or substitute an easy, gentle exercise.

WEEK 3

	SUN	MON	TUE	WED	THU	FRI	SAT	
								Resting Pulse Rate
	35	20	Free	35	30	30	30	Walking Time
	70	60	X	70	60	70	60	W. H. R.
	F	F	X	M	F	H	F	Course Profile
			X					Air Temperature
								Notes/Comments

WEEK 4

	SUN	MON	TUE	WED	THU	FRI	SAT	
								Resting Pulse Rate
	40	25	Free	40	30	35	Free	Walking Time
	70	60	X	70	60	70	X	W.H. R.
	F	F	X	M	F	M	X	Course Profile
			X					Air Temperature
								Notes/Comments

Under "Course Profile": F = Flat, H = Hilly, M = Mixed

My Working Heart Rate
60% = _____ bpm
70% = _____ bpm
80% = _____ bpm

WEEKS 5 – 8

THE TOP-OF-THE-PYRAMID PROGRAM WEEKS 5-8

WEEK 5

	SUN	MON	TUE	WED	THU	FRI	SAT
Resting Pulse Rate							
Walking Time	30	20	Free	30	30	30	Bike
W. H. R.	70	60	X	70	60	70	X
Course Profile	F	F	X	F	F	F	X
Air Temperature			X				X
Notes/Comments							

WEEK 6

	SUN	MON	TUE	WED	THU	FRI	SAT
Resting Pulse Rate							
Walking Time	35	20	Free	35	30	30	30
W.H. R.	80	60	X	70	60	70	60
Course Profile	F	F	X	F	F	F	F
Air Temperature			X				
Notes/Comments							

Under ''Course Profile'': F = Flat, H = Hilly, M = Mixed

REMEMBER: When the schedule calls for a Hilly Course, it does not mean radical hills; a 3 or 4% grade is more than enough.

WEEK 7

	SUN	MON	TUE	WED	THU	FRI	SAT	
								Resting Pulse Rate
	40	25	Free	40	30	35	Free	Walking Time
	80	60	X	70	60	70	X	W. H. R.
	F	F	X	F	F	M	X	Course Profile
		X					X	Air Temperature
								Notes/Comments

WEEK 8

	SUN	MON	TUE	WED	THU	FRI	SAT	
								Resting Pulse Rate
	45	30	Free	45	30	40	30	Walking Time
	80	60	X	70	60	70	60	W.H. R.
	M	F	X	H	F	F	F	Course Profile
		X						Air Temperature
								Notes/Comments

Under "Course Profile": F = Flat, H = Hilly, M = Mixed

My Working Heart Rate
60% = ____ bpm
70% = ____ bpm
80% = ____ bpm

WEEKS 9 — 12

WEEK 9

	SUN	MON	TUE	WED	THU	FRI	SAT
Resting Pulse Rate							
Walking Time	35	20	Free	35	30	30	30
W. H. R.	80	60	X	70	60	70	60
Course Profile	M	F	X	F	F	F	F
Air Temperature			X				
Notes/Comments							

WEEK 10

	SUN	MON	TUE	WED	THU	FRI	SAT
Resting Pulse Rate							
Walking Time	40	25	Free	40	30	35	Free
W.H. R.	80	60	X	70	60	70	X
Course Profile	F	F	X	F	F	F	X
Air Temperature			X				X
Notes/Comments							

Under "Course Profile": F = Flat, H = Hilly, M = Mixed

REMEMBER: When you come to an intersection and must stop, take the opportunity to check your Working Heart Rate.

WEEK 11

	SUN	MON	TUE	WED	THU	FRI	SAT	
								Resting Pulse Rate
Walking Time	45	30	Free	45	35	45	30	Walking Time
W. H. R.	80	60	X	70	60	70	60	W. H. R.
Course Profile	F	F	X	F	F	M	F	Course Profile
Air Temperature			X					Air Temperature
Notes/Comments								Notes/Comments

WEEK 12

	SUN	MON	TUE	WED	THU	FRI	SAT	
								Resting Pulse Rate
Walking Time	60	35	Free	50	40	50	30	Walking Time
W.H. R.	70	60	X	70	60	70	60	W.H. R.
Course Profile	M	F	X	H	F	F	F	Course Profile
Air Temperature			X					Air Temperature
Notes/Comments								Notes/Comments

Under "Course Profile": F = Flat, H = Hilly, M = Mixed

WEEKS 13 — 16

THE TOP-OF-THE-PYRAMID PROGRAM   WEEKS 13-16

WEEK 13

	SUN	MON	TUE	WED	THU	FRI	SAT
Resting Pulse Rate							
Walking Time	35	20	Free	30	30	30	Bike
W. H. R.	70	60	X	70	60	70	X
Course Profile	F	F	X	F	F	F	X
Air Temperature			X				X
Notes/Comments							

WEEK 14

	SUN	MON	TUE	WED	THU	FRI	SAT
Resting Pulse Rate							
Walking Time	35	25	Free	40	30	30	30
W.H. R.	80	60	X	70	60	70	60
Course Profile	F	F	X	F	F	F	F
Air Temperature			X				
Notes/Comments							

Under "Course Profile": **F** = Flat, **H** = Hilly, **M** = Mixed

REMEMBER: If, after beginning this program, you find it is too much too soon, drop back to the 90-Day program.

WEEK 15

SUN	MON	TUE	WED	THU	FRI	SAT	
							Resting Pulse Rate
40	25	Free	40	30	35	Free	Walking Time
80	60	X	70	60	70	X	W. H. R.
F	F	X	F	F	M	X	Course Profile
		X				X	Air Temperature
							Notes/Comments

WEEK 16

SUN	MON	TUE	WED	THU	FRI	SAT	
							Resting Pulse Rate
45	30	Free	45	35	45	30	Walking Time
80	60	X	70	60	70	60	W.H. R.
M	F	X	H	F	F	F	Course Profile
		X					Air Temperature
							Notes/Comments

Under "Course Profile": F = Flat, H = Hilly, M = Mixed

My Working Heart Rate
60% = _____ bpm
70% = _____ bpm
80% = _____ bpm

WEEKS 17— 20

WEEK 17

	SUN	MON	TUE	WED	THU	FRI	SAT
Resting Pulse Rate							
Walking Time	35	25	Free	40	30	30	30
W. H. R.	80	60	X	70	60	70	60
Course Profile	F	F	X	F	F	F	F
Air Temperature			X				
Notes/Comments							

WEEK 18

	SUN	MON	TUE	WED	THU	FRI	SAT
Resting Pulse Rate							
Walking Time	40	25	Free	40	30	35	Bike
W.H. R.	80	60	X	70	60	70	X
Course Profile	F	F	X	F	F	F	X
Air Temperature			X				X
Notes/Comments							

Under "Course Profile": F=Flat, H=Hilly, M=Mixed

REMEMBER:
Even though there is no reminder to do Warm-Up and Cool-Down exercises, they should be part of every workout.

WEEK 19

SUN	MON	TUE	WED	THU	FRI	SAT	
							Resting Pulse Rate
45	39	Free	45	35	45	30	Walking Time
80	60	X	70	60	70	60	W. H. R.
F	F	X	F	F	M	X	Course Profile
		X					Air Temperature
							Notes/Comments

WEEK 20

SUN	MON	TUE	WED	THU	FRI	SAT	
							Resting Pulse Rate
70	40	Free	45	40	45	30	Walking Time
70	60	X	80	60	70	60	W.H. R.
M	F	X	H	F	F	F	Course Profile
		X					Air Temperature
							Notes/Comments

Under "Course Profile": F = Flat, H = Hilly, M = Mixed

<table>
<tr><td colspan="2" rowspan="3">**My Working Heart Rate**

60% = ___ bpm
70% = ___ bpm
80% = ___ bpm</td></tr>
</table>

WEEKS 21— 24

WEEK

21

	SUN	MON	TUE	WED	THU	FRI	SAT
Resting Pulse Rate							
Walking Time	40	25	Free	40	30	35	Free
W. H. R.	80	60	X	70	60	70	X
Course Profile	F	F	X	F	F	F	X
Air Temperature			X				X
Notes/Comments							

WEEK

22

	SUN	MON	TUE	WED	THU	FRI	SAT
Resting Pulse Rate							
Walking Time	45	30	Free	45	35	45	30
W.H. R.	80	60	X	70	60	70	60
Course Profile	F	F	X	F	F	F	F
Air Temperature			X				
Notes/Comments							

THE TOP-OF-THE-PYRAMID PROGRAM   WEEKS 21-24

Under "Course Profile": **F** = Flat, **H** = Hilly, **M** = Mixed

REMEMBER: The more ambitious your program becomes, the less chance you will be able to do it with training partners. Depend upon yourself.

WEEK 23

	SUN	MON	TUE	WED	THU	FRI	SAT	
								Resting Pulse Rate
	70	40	Free	45	40	45	Bike	Walking Time
	70	60	X	80	60	70	X	W. H. R.
	F	F	X	F	F	M	X	Course Profile
			X				X	Air Temperature
								Notes/Comments

WEEK 24

	SUN	MON	TUE	WED	THU	FRI	SAT	
								Resting Pulse Rate
	75	45	Free	60	45	45	40	Walking Time
	70	60	X	70	60	70	60	W.H. R.
	M	F	X	H	F	F	F	Course Profile
			X					Air Temperature
								Notes/Comments

Under "Course Profile": F=Flat, H=Hilly, M=Mixed

My Working Heart Rate
60% = _____ bpm
70% = _____ bpm
80% = _____ bpm

WEEKS 25 — 28

WEEK   25

	SUN	MON	TUE	WED	THU	FRI	SAT
Resting Pulse Rate							
Walking Time	35	25	Free	40	30	30	30
W. H. R.	80	60	X	70	60	70	60
Course Profile	F	F	X	F	F	F	F
Air Temperature			X				
Notes/Comments							

WEEK   26

	SUN	MON	TUE	WED	THU	FRI	SAT
Resting Pulse Rate							
Walking Time	40	30	Free	45	30	35	Free
W.H. R.	80	60	X	70	60	70	X
Course Profile	F	F	X	F	F	F	X
Air Temperature			X				X
Notes/Comments							

Under ''Course Profile'': F = Flat, H = Hilly, M = Mixed

REMEMBER: If your Resting Pulse Rate rises by more than 5 points above normal, take it easy in your exercising that day.

WEEK 27

SUN	MON	TUE	WED	THU	FRI	SAT	
							Resting Pulse Rate
45	30	Free	45	35	45	30	Walking Time
80	60	X	70	60	70	60	W. H. R.
F	F	X	F	F	M	F	Course Profile
		X					Air Temperature
							Notes/Comments

WEEK 28

SUN	MON	TUE	WED	THU	FRI	SAT	
							Resting Pulse Rate
70	40	Free	45	40	45	30	Walking Time
70	60	X	80	60	70	60	W.H. R.
M	F	X	H	F	F	F	Course Profile
		X					Air Temperature
							Notes/Comments

Under "Course Profile": F = Flat, H = Hilly, M = Mixed

My Working Heart Rate
60% = _____ bpm
70% = _____ bpm
80% = _____ bpm

WEEKS 29 — 32

WEEK 29

	SUN	MON	TUE	WED	THU	FRI	SAT
Resting Pulse Rate							
Walking Time	40	30	Free	45	30	35	Free
W. H. R.	80	60	X	70	60	70	X
Course Profile	F	F	X	F	F	F	X
Air Temperature			X				X
Notes/Comments							

WEEK 30

	SUN	MON	TUE	WED	THU	FRI	SAT
Resting Pulse Rate							
Walking Time	45	30	Free	45	35	45	30
W.H. R.	80	60	X	70	60	70	60
Course Profile	F	F	X	F	F	F	F
Air Temperature			X				
Notes/Comments							

Under "Course Profile": F = Flat, H = Hilly, M = Mixed

REMEMBER: Do not push your walking pace beyond the recommended W.H.R. for that particular day. Patience always wins out.

WEEK 31

SUN	MON	TUE	WED	THU	FRI	SAT	
							Resting Pulse Rate
70	40	Free	45	40	45	Bike	Walking Time
70	60	X	80	60	70	X	W. H. R.
F	F	X	F	F	M	X	Course Profile
		X				X	Air Temperature
							Notes/Comments

WEEK 32

SUN	MON	TUE	WED	THU	FRI	SAT	
							Resting Pulse Rate
75	45	Free	60	45	45	40	Walking Time
70	60	X	70	60	70	60	W.H. R.
M	F	X	H	F	F	F	Course Profile
		X					Air Temperature
							Notes/Comments

Under "Course Profile": F = Flat, H = Hilly, M = Mixed

WEEKS 33 — 36

THE TOP-OF-THE-PYRAMID PROGRAM   WEEKS 33-36

WEEK 33

	SUN	MON	TUE	WED	THU	FRI	SAT
Resting Pulse Rate							
Walking Time	45	30	Free	45	35	45	30
W. H. R.	80	60	X	70	60	70	60
Course Profile	F	F	X	F	F	F	F
Air Temperature			X				
Notes/Comments							

WEEK 34

	SUN	MON	TUE	WED	THU	FRI	SAT
Resting Pulse Rate							
Walking Time	70	40	Free	45	40	45	Free
W.H. R.	70	60	X	80	60	70	X
Course Profile	F	F	X	F	F	F	X
Air Temperature			X				X
Notes/Comments							

Under "Course Profile": F = Flat, H = Hilly, M = Mixed

REMEMBER: Do not be afraid to jot down random thoughts and impressions under Notes/Comments — it is your daily diary.

WEEK 35

SUN	MON	TUE	WED	THU	FRI	SAT	
							Resting Pulse Rate
75	45	Free	60	45	45	40	Walking Time
70	60	X	70	60	70	60	W. H. R.
F	F	X	F	F	M	F	Course Profile
		X					Air Temperature
							Notes/Comments

WEEK 36

SUN	MON	TUE	WED	THU	FRI	SAT	
							Resting Pulse Rate
90	45	Free	60	45	45	45	Walking Time
70	60	X	80	60	70	60	W.H. R.
M	F	X	H	F	F	F	Course Profile
		X					Air Temperature
							Notes/Comments

Under "Course Profile": F = Flat, H = Hilly, M = Mixed

My Working Heart Rate
60% = _____ bpm
70% = _____ bpm
80% = _____ bpm

WEEKS 37 — 40

WEEK 37

	SUN	MON	TUE	WED	THU	FRI	SAT
Resting Pulse Rate							
Walking Time	70	40	Free	45	40	45	Bike
W. H. R.	70	60	X	80	60	70	X
Course Profile	F	F	X	F	F	F	X
Air Temperature			X				X
Notes/Comments							

WEEK 38

	SUN	MON	TUE	WED	THU	FRI	SAT
Resting Pulse Rate							
Walking Time	75	45	Free	60	45	45	40
W.H. R.	70	60	X	70	60	70	60
Course Profile	F	F	X	F	F	F	F
Air Temperature			X				
Notes/Comments							

Under "Course Profile": F = Flat, H = Hilly, M = Mixed

REMEMBER:
If the outdoor temperature is extremely hostile (either too hot or cold), be creative: move inside and walk in your local mall.

WEEK 39

SUN	MON	TUE	WED	THU	FRI	SAT	
							Resting Pulse Rate
90	45	Free	60	45	45	45	Walking Time
70	60	X	80	60	70	60	W. H. R.
F	F	X	F	F	M	F	Course Profile
		X					Air Temperature
							Notes/Comments

WEEK 40

SUN	MON	TUE	WED	THU	FRI	SAT	
							Resting Pulse Rate
90	50	Free	60	45	45	45	Walking Time
80	60	X	80	70	80	60	W.H. R.
M	F	X	H	F	F	F	Course Profile
		X					Air Temperature
							Notes/Comments

Under "Course Profile": F = Flat, H = Hilly, M = Mixed

WEEKS 41 — 44

THE TOP-OF-THE-PYRAMID PROGRAM   WEEKS 41-44

WEEK 41

	SUN	MON	TUE	WED	THU	FRI	SAT
Resting Pulse Rate							
Walking Time	40	30	Free	45	30	35	Free
W. H. R.	80	60	X	70	60	70	X
Course Profile	F	F	X	F	F	F	X
Air Temperature			X				X
Notes/Comments							

WEEK 42

	SUN	MON	TUE	WED	THU	FRI	SAT
Resting Pulse Rate							
Walking Time	30	20	Free	30	30	30	Free
W.H. R.	70	60	X	70	60	70	X
Course Profile	F	F	X	F	F	M	X
Air Temperature			X				X
Notes/Comments							

Under "Course Profile": F = Flat, H = Hilly, M = Mixed

REMEMBER:

WEEK 43

SUN	MON	TUE	WED	THU	FRI	SAT	
							Resting Pulse Rate
120	30	Free	60	45	45	Free	Walking Time
70	60	X	70	60	70	X	W. H. R.
M	F	X	H	F	F	X	Course Profile
		X				X	Air Temperature
							Notes/Comments

WEEK 44

SUN	MON	TUE	WED	THU	FRI	SAT	
							Resting Pulse Rate
25	20	Free	25	30	25	Free	Walking Time
70	60	X	70	60	70	X	W.H. R.
F	F	X	F	F	F	X	Course Profile
		X				X	Air Temperature
							Notes/Comments

Under "Course Profile": F = Flat, H = Hilly, M = Mixed

My Working Heart Rate
60% = ____ bpm
70% = ____ bpm
80% = ____ bpm

WEEK 45

	SUN	MON	TUE	WED	THU	FRI	SAT
Resting Pulse Rate							
Walking Time	25	20	Free	25	30	25	Free
W. H. R.	70	60	X	70	60	70	X
Course Profile	F	F	X	F	F	F	X
Air Temperature			X				X
Notes/Comments							

WEEK 46

	SUN	MON	TUE	WED	THU	FRI	SAT
Resting Pulse Rate							
Walking Time	30	20	Free	30	30	30	Bike
W.H. R.	70	60	X	70	60	70	X
Course Profile	F	F	X	F	F	F	X
Air Temperature			X				X
Notes/Comments							

Under ''Course Profile'': F = Flat, H = Hilly, M = Mixed

THE TOP-OF-THE-PYRAMID PROGRAM   WEEKS 45-48

REMEMBER: When you are walking, keep your body erect and walk with a smile — and with the authority of a person with a destination in mind.

WEEK 47

SUN	MON	TUE	WED	THU	FRI	SAT	
							Resting Pulse Rate
25	20	Free	25	30	25	Free	Walking Time
70	60	X	70	60	70	X	W. H. R.
F	F	X	F	F	F	X	Course Profile
		X				X	Air Temperature
							Notes/Comments

WEEK 48

SUN	MON	TUE	WED	THU	FRI	SAT	
							Resting Pulse Rate
30	20	Free	30	30	30	Bike	Walking Time
70	60	X	70	60	70	X	W.H. R.
F	F	X	F	F	F	X	Course Profile
		X				X	Air Temperature
							Notes/Comments

Under ''Course Profile'': F = Flat, H = Hilly, M = Mixed

My Working Heart Rate
60% = ＿＿ bpm
70% = ＿＿ bpm
80% = ＿＿ bpm

WEEKS 49 — 52

WEEK 49

	SUN	MON	TUE	WED	THU	FRI	SAT
Resting Pulse Rate							
Walking Time	30	20	Free	30	30	30	Free
W. H. R.	70	60	X	70	60	70	X
Course Profile	F	F	X	F	F	M	X
Air Temperature			X				X
Notes/Comments							

WEEK 50

	SUN	MON	TUE	WED	THU	FRI	SAT
Resting Pulse Rate							
Walking Time	35	25	Free	40	30	30	30
W.H. R.	80	60	X	70	60	70	60
Course Profile	M	F	X	F	F	F	F
Air Temperature			X				
Notes/Comments							

Under "Course Profile": F = Flat, H = Hilly, M = Mixed

REMEMBER: Take it easy when walking after a heavy meal. Much of your blood has been diverted from the working muscles to the stomach.

WEEK 51

SUN	MON	TUE	WED	THU	FRI	SAT	
							Resting Pulse Rate
30	25	Free	30	30	30	Bike	Walking Time
70	60	X	70	60	70	X	W. H. R.
F	F	X	F	F	M	X	Course Profile
	X					X	Air Temperature
							Notes/Comments

WEEK 52

SUN	MON	TUE	WED	THU	FRI	SAT	
							Resting Pulse Rate
35	25	Free	40	30	30	30	Walking Time
80	60	X	70	60	70	60	W.H. R.
M	F	X	M	F	F	F	Course Profile
	X						Air Temperature
							Notes/Comments

Under "Course Profile": F = Flat, H = Hilly, M = Mixed

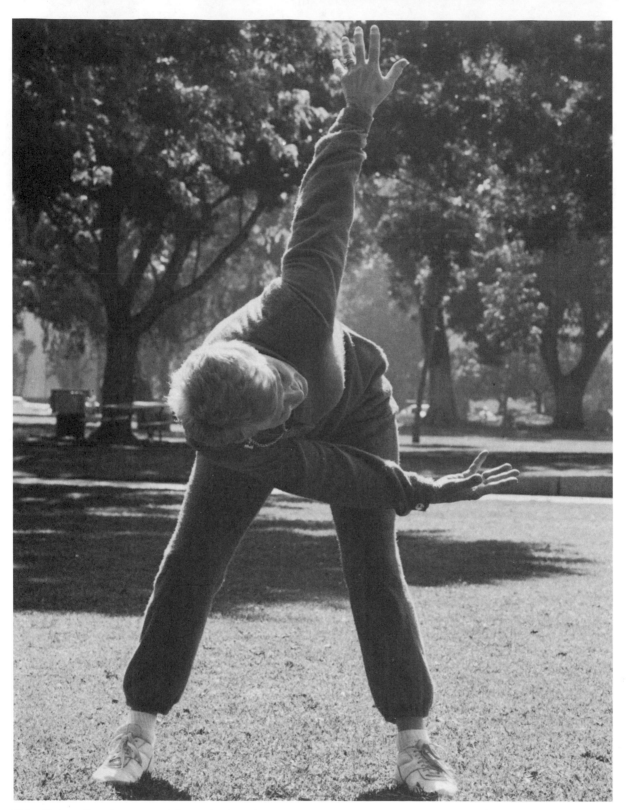

The Great Outdoors—Although the photos in which the warm-up and cool-down exercises are shown were shot indoors, that doesn't mean that the exercises must be done indoors. When the weather is pleasant, I like to stay outside while I do my cool-down exercises. It extends the good feeling of being outdoors that much longer, and can make you feel so good it's almost like a good therapy session.

Chapter 11

The Lifetime Program Of Walking For Health, Fitness & Weight Control

*"Walking is the best possible exercise.
Habituate yourself to walk very far."*
—Thomas Jefferson

The reason most diets work only temporarily is because they are not designed for long-term use and they are either boring or difficult to maintain.

The same could be said for exercise programs: the more difficult or monotonous, the more likely a person is to abandon it. That's why I like to think that we all should go on a "way of life," not only in our physical activities but in our nutritional habits.

The "way of life" program that follows features four progressively more difficult walking programs (designated A, B, C, and D) based on walking time and Working Heart Rate. The A, B, C, and D Working Heart Rate percentages outline the effort that you are putting out.

These programs are designed to begin where you left off at either Chapter 9 or 10 and are structured with flexibility that heads off boredom by generating variety. The program is based on a 24-week cycle rather than a 26-week cycle. By doing this you will vary your program. For instance, what you do at Week 7 in the first cycle will be done at a different time of the year from Week 7 in the next 24-week cycle and so on, insuring seasonal variety. After completing each 24-week cycle, you should be able to move on to the next 24 weeks with relative ease.

Please remember that each year we grow a year older. Consequently, each year you should return to the end of Chapter 5 to recalculate your Working Heart Rates (W.H.R.). Then place your new W.H.R.s in the boxes provided in the upper left of each month's programs.

Remember to do your Warm-Up and Cool-Down exercises each time you do a workout.

And let's all keep on walking to fitness and health!

My Working Heart Rate
60% = _____ bpm
70% = _____ bpm
80% = _____ bpm

WEEKS 1 — 4

WEEK 1

		SUN	MON	TUE	WED	THU	FRI	SAT
Resting Pulse Rate								
Walking Time	A	35	25	FREE	40	30	30	FREE
	B	35	25	FREE	40	30	30	FREE
	C	40	25	FREE	40	35	30	30
	D	40	30	FREE	45	35	30	35
W. H. R.	A	80	60	X	70	60	70	X
	B	80	60	X	70	60	70	X
	C	80	60	X	70	60	70	60
	D	80	70	X	70	60	70	60
Notes/Comments								

WEEK 2

		SUN	MON	TUE	WED	THU	FRI	SAT
Resting Pulse Rate								
Walking Time	A	40	25	FREE	45	30	30	30
	B	40	30	FREE	45	35	35	35
	C	45	30	FREE	50	35	35	35
	D	45	30	FREE	50	35	35	35
W.H. R.	A	70	60	X	70	60	70	60
	B	70	60	X	70	60	70	60
	C	70	60	X	70	60	70	60
	D	70	60	X	70	60	70	60
Notes/Comments								

REMEMBER: Each year, recalculate your W.H.R. by repeating the calculations outlined at the end of chapter 5.

WEEK   3

SUN	MON	TUE	WED	THU	FRI	SAT		
								Resting Pulse Rate
45	30	FREE	45	35	30	35	A	
50	30	FREE	45	35	35	35	B	Walking Time
60	30	FREE	45	35	40	35	C	
65	30	FREE	50	35	45	35	D	
70	60	X	70	70	70	60	A	
70	60	X	70	70	70	60	B	W. H. R.
70	60	X	70	70	70	60	C	
70	60	X	70	70	70	60	D	
								Notes/Comments

WEEK   4

SUN	MON	TUE	WED	THU	FRI	SAT		
								Resting Pulse Rate
40	30	FREE	40	30	30	FREE	A	
45	30	FREE	45	35	35	FREE	B	Walking Time
50	30	FREE	45	35	35	FREE	C	
55	30	FREE	45	35	35	FREE	D	
70	60	X	70	60	70	X	A	
70	60	X	70	60	70	X	B	W.H. R.
70	60	X	70	60	70	X	C	
70	60	X	70	60	70	X	D	
								Notes/Comments

My Working Heart Rate
60% = ____ bpm
70% = ____ bpm
80% = ____ bpm

WEEKS 5 — 8

WEEK						**5**
SUN	**MON**	**TUE**	**WED**	**THU**	**FRI**	**SAT**

		SUN	MON	TUE	WED	THU	FRI	SAT
Resting Pulse Rate								
Walking Time	A	40	30	FREE	45	30	30	30
	B	45	30	FREE	50	35	40	30
	C	50	30	FREE	55	35	40	30
	D	55	30	FREE	60	40	45	30
W. H. R.	A	80	60	X	70	60	70	60
	B	80	60	X	70	60	70	60
	C	80	60	X	70	60	70	60
	D	80	60	X	70	60	70	60
Notes/Comments								

WEEK						**6**
SUN	**MON**	**TUE**	**WED**	**THU**	**FRI**	**SAT**

		SUN	MON	TUE	WED	THU	FRI	SAT
Resting Pulse Rate								
Walking Time	A	45	30	FREE	45	30	30	FREE
	B	50	30	FREE	50	35	35	FREE
	C	55	30	FREE	55	35	35	30
	D	60	30	FREE	60	40	40	30
W.H. R.	A	70	60	X	70	60	70	X
	B	70	60	X	70	60	70	X
	C	70	60	X	70	60	70	60
	D	70	60	X	70	60	70	60
Notes/Comments								

REMEMBER: The length of time for each indicated walk begins when your heart rate rises to the percentage indicated.

WEEK 7

SUN	MON	TUE	WED	THU	FRI	SAT		
								Resting Pulse Rate
45	30	FREE	45	30	35	30	A	
50	30	FREE	50	35	40	35	B	Walking Time
55	30	FREE	55	35	45	35	C	
60	30	FREE	60	40	50	30	D	
80	60	X	70	60	70	60	A	
80	60	X	70	60	70	60	B	W. H. R.
80	60	X	70	60	70	60	C	
80	60	X	70	60	70	60	D	
								Notes/Comments

WEEK 8

SUN	MON	TUE	WED	THU	FRI	SAT		
								Resting Pulse Rate
45	30	FREE	40	30	30	FREE	A	
50	30	FREE	45	35	35	FREE	B	Walking Time
55	30	FREE	50	35	40	FREE	C	
60	30	FREE	55	40	45	FREE	D	
70	60	X	70	60	70	X	A	
70	60	X	70	60	70	X	B	W.H. R.
70	60	X	70	60	70	X	C	
70	60	X	70	60	70	X	D	
								Notes/Comments

My Working Heart Rate
60% = _____ bpm
70% = _____ bpm
80% = _____ bpm

WEEKS 9 — 12

WEEK 9

		SUN	MON	TUE	WED	THU	FRI	SAT
Resting Pulse Rate								
Walking Time	A	50	30	FREE	40	30	30	30
	B	60	30	FREE	45	35	35	30
	C	70	30	FREE	50	35	40	30
	D	75	30	FREE	55	40	45	30
W. H. R.	A	80	60	X	70	60	70	60
	B	80	60	X	70	60	70	60
	C	80	60	X	70	60	70	60
	D	80	60	X	70	60	70	60
Notes/Comments								

WEEK 10

		SUN	MON	TUE	WED	THU	FRI	SAT
Resting Pulse Rate								
Walking Time	A	60	30	FREE	45	30	35	FREE
	B	70	30	FREE	50	35	35	FREE
	C	75	30	FREE	55	35	40	30
	D	80	30	FREE	60	40	45	30
W.H. R.	A	70	60	X	60	60	70	X
	B	70	60	X	60	60	70	X
	C	70	60	X	60	60	70	60
	D	70	60	X	60	60	70	60
Notes/Comments								

REMEMBER:
Do your Warm-Up and Cool-Down exercises before and after each workout. Doing this helps prevent injuries.

WEEK 11

SUN	MON	TUE	WED	THU	FRI	SAT		
								Resting Pulse Rate
60	30	FREE	45	30	40	30	A	
70	30	FREE	50	35	45	30	B	Walking Time
75	30	FREE	55	35	50	30	C	
80	30	FREE	60	40	55	30	D	
70	60	X	70	60	70	60	A	
70	60	X	70	60	70	60	B	W. H. R.
70	60	X	70	60	70	60	C	
70	60	X	70	60	70	60	D	
								Notes/Comments

WEEK 12

SUN	MON	TUE	WED	THU	FRI	SAT		
								Resting Pulse Rate
50	30	FREE	40	30	30	FREE	A	
60	30	FREE	45	35	35	FREE	B	Walking Time
70	30	FREE	50	35	40	30	C	
80	30	FREE	55	40	45	30	D	
70	60	X	60	60	70	X	A	
70	60	X	60	60	70	X	B	W.H. R.
70	60	X	60	60	70	60	C	
70	60	X	60	60	70	60	D	
								Notes/Comments

My Working Heart Rate
60% = ____ bpm
70% = ____ bpm
80% = ____ bpm

WEEKS 13 — 16

WEEK 13

		SUN	MON	TUE	WED	THU	FRI	SAT
Resting Pulse Rate								
Walking Time	A	60	30	FREE	45	30	30	30
	B	60	35	FREE	50	35	35	30
	C	70	35	FREE	55	35	40	30
	D	75	35	FREE	60	40	45	30
W. H. R.	A	70	60	X	70	60	70	60
	B	70	60	X	70	60	70	60
	C	70	60	X	70	60	70	60
	D	70	60	X	70	60	70	60
Notes/Comments								

WEEK 14

		SUN	MON	TUE	WED	THU	FRI	SAT
Resting Pulse Rate								
Walking Time	A	60	30	FREE	45	30	40	FREE
	B	70	35	FREE	50	35	45	FREE
	C	75	35	FREE	55	35	50	30
	D	80	35	FREE	60	40	55	30
W.H. R.	A	80	60	X	70	60	70	X
	B	80	60	X	70	60	70	X
	C	80	60	X	70	60	70	60
	D	80	60	X	70	60	70	60
Notes/Comments								

REMEMBER: Make every attempt to eat a balanced diet, and make it a point to drink plenty of water.

WEEK 15

SUN	MON	TUE	WED	THU	FRI	SAT		
								Resting Pulse Rate
60	30	FREE	45	30	45	30	A	
70	35	FREE	50	35	50	30	B	Walking Time
75	35	FREE	55	35	55	30	C	
80	35	FREE	60	40	60	30	D	
80	60	X	80	60	70	60	A	
80	60	X	80	60	70	60	B	W. H. R.
80	60	X	80	60	70	60	C	
80	60	X	80	60	70	60	D	
								Notes/Comments

WEEK 16

SUN	MON	TUE	WED	THU	FRI	SAT		
								Resting Pulse Rate
60	30	FREE	45	30	40	FREE	A	
70	35	FREE	50	35	45	FREE	B	Walking Time
75	35	FREE	55	35	50	30	C	
80	35	FREE	60	40	55	30	D	
70	60	X	70	60	70	X	A	
70	60	X	70	60	70	X	B	W.H. R.
70	60	X	70	60	70	60	C	
70	60	X	70	60	70	60	D	
								Notes/Comments

My Working Heart Rate
60% = ____ bpm
70% = ____ bpm
80% = ____ bpm

WEEKS 17 — 20

WEEK — 17

		SUN	MON	TUE	WED	THU	FRI	SAT
Resting Pulse Rate								
Walking Time	A	60	30	FREE	45	30	40	30
	B	70	35	FREE	50	40	45	30
	C	75	35	FREE	55	40	50	30
	D	80	35	FREE	60	40	55	30
W. H. R.	A	80	60	X	70	60	70	60
	B	80	60	X	70	60	70	60
	C	80	60	X	70	60	70	60
	D	80	60	X	70	60	70	60
Notes/Comments								

WEEK — 18

		SUN	MON	TUE	WED	THU	FRI	SAT
Resting Pulse Rate								
Walking Time	A	60	30	FREE	45	30	40	FREE
	B	70	35	FREE	50	35	45	FREE
	C	75	35	FREE	55	35	50	30
	D	80	35	FREE	60	40	55	30
W.H. R.	A	80	60	X	80	60	70	X
	B	80	60	X	80	60	70	X
	C	80	60	X	80	60	70	60
	D	80	60	X	80	60	70	60
Notes/Comments								

REMEMBER:

WEEK   19

SUN	MON	TUE	WED	THU	FRI	SAT		
								Resting Pulse Rate
60	30	FREE	45	30	45	40	A	
70	35	FREE	50	35	50	40	B	Walking Time
75	35	FREE	55	35	55	40	C	
80	35	FREE	60	40	60	40	D	
80	60	X	80	60	70	60	A	
80	60	X	80	60	70	60	B	W. H. R.
80	60	X	80	60	70	60	C	
80	60	X	80	60	70	60	D	
								Notes/Comments

WEEK   20

SUN	MON	TUE	WED	THU	FRI	SAT		
								Resting Pulse Rate
45	30	FREE	45	30	45	FREE	A	
50	35	FREE	50	35	50	FREE	B	Walking Time
55	35	FREE	55	35	55	35	C	
60	35	FREE	60	40	60	35	D	
80	60	X	70	60	60	X	A	
80	60	X	70	60	60	X	B	W.H. R.
80	60	X	70	60	60	60	C	
80	60	X	70	60	60	60	D	
								Notes/Comments

WEEKS 21 — 24

WEEK 21

		SUN	MON	TUE	WED	THU	FRI	SAT
Resting Pulse Rate								
Walking Time	A	45	30	FREE	45	30	40	30
	B	50	30	FREE	45	35	45	30
	C	55	35	FREE	50	35	50	30
	D	60	35	FREE	50	40	50	30
W. H. R.	A	80	60	X	70	60	50	60
	B	80	60	X	70	60	60	60
	C	80	60	X	70	60	60	60
	D	80	60	X	70	60	60	60
Notes/Comments								

WEEK 22

		SUN	MON	TUE	WED	THU	FRI	SAT
Resting Pulse Rate								
Walking Time	A	40	30	FREE	40	30	40	FREE
	B	45	35	FREE	45	30	40	FREE
	C	50	35	FREE	45	30	40	FREE
	D	50	35	FREE	45	30	40	30
W.H. R.	A	80	60	X	70	60	60	X
	B	80	60	X	70	60	60	X
	C	80	60	X	70	60	60	X
	D	80	60	X	70	60	60	60
Notes/Comments								

REMEMBER: Lead others to walking — not by telling them how to do it, but by showing them what good it does for you.

WEEK 23

SUN	MON	TUE	WED	THU	FRI	SAT		
								Resting Pulse Rate
45	30	FREE	40	30	35	30	A	
45	30	FREE	40	30	35	30	B	Walking Time
45	30	FREE	40	30	35	30	C	
45	30	FREE	40	30	35	30	D	
70	60	X	70	60	70	60	A	
80	60	X	70	60	70	60	B	W. H. R.
80	60	X	70	60	70	60	C	
80	60	X	70	60	70	60	D	
								Notes/Comments

WEEK 24

SUN	MON	TUE	WED	THU	FRI	SAT		
								Resting Pulse Rate
40	30	FREE	40	30	30	FREE	A	
40	30	FREE	40	30	30	FREE	B	Walking Time
40	30	FREE	40	30	30	FREE	C	
40	30	FREE	40	30	30	FREE	D	
70	60	X	70	60	70	X	A	
70	60	X	70	60	70	X	B	W.H. R.
70	60	X	70	60	70	X	C	
70	60	X	70	60	70	X	D	
								Notes/Comments

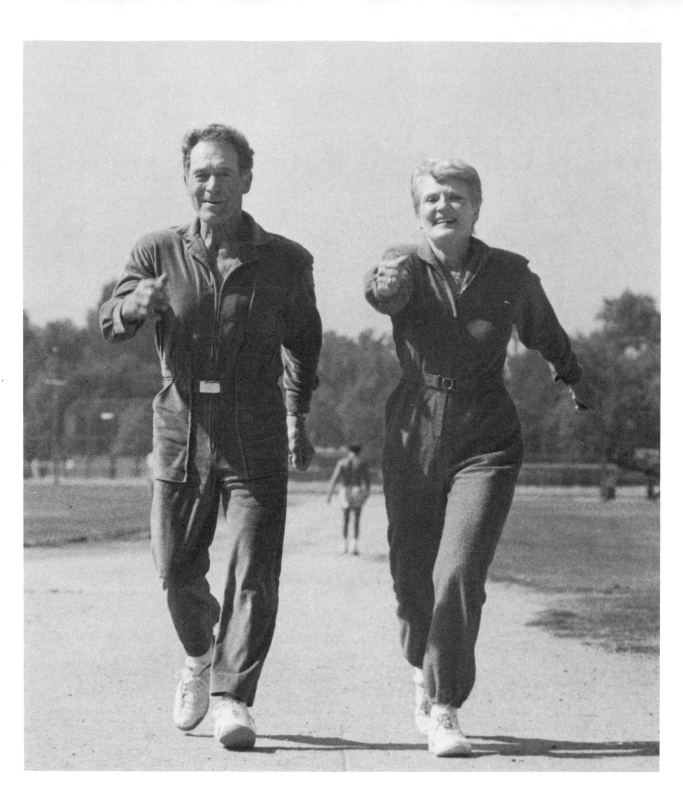

Get on Track—Although the courses outlined in Chapter 4 are set up as though you're doing all your workouts in and around your neighborhood, don't be afraid to improvise. If there is a nice park you can go to to do your Dynastriding, why not take a bus or drive to it and do your workout on the park trails and paths? Or go to the local high school or college track and do your Dynastriding around the track at least once a week? You'll have no pesky traffic to worry about at either the park or at the local track. There is almost no place in the world that is off limits to the energetic Dynastrider!

Chapter 12
Physical Challenges

"Come, you and I must walk a turn together."
Henry VIII Act V, Scene 1
—William Shakespeare

At several places in this book I've made the statement that virtually anyone can walk. This is, of course, true. Walking is one of the most basic of human actions. However, there are some people for whom the act of walking is very difficult and even painful, and there are other people who are simply unable to walk because of physical limitations.

Certainly, no one exercise program is right for 100% of the people on this planet. There are *always* exceptions.

While some people would not be able to benefit from my walking program, they could benefit from applying some of the principles to an exercise program adapted to their limitations, no matter how modest it might be.

I've seen people with even the most severe disabilities enrich their lives by beginning—and sticking with—an exercise program.

For instance, Bob Wieland, a Vietnam veteran who lost both legs in combat, built his body up to the point that he was able to walk across America on his hands. He literally made his arms his legs and his hands his feet. He is also a four-time world champion in the bench press against able-bodied men.

One group of people limited in their exercise horizons that is numerous among the over-50 age group is people suffering from severe arthritis. For arthritis sufferers nearly every movement can be painful. Yet, ironically, certain exercises can help alleviate some of the pain and discomfort of arthritis. Regular exercise can help slow the onset of arthritis and can mediate its impact when it does come. Of course, if you've never exercised but suffer from serious arthritis, it is going to be uncomfortable at first.

There are ways to exercise while minimizing the pain of arthritis, however.

Perhaps the best program I know of is one formulated by a long-time arthritis sufferer, Dvera Berson of Brooklyn. By the time she was 60 years old, she had been suffering for six years. She was diagnosed as having rheumatoid arthritis and osteoarthritis, osteoporosis and cervical spondylosis deformans. Dvera was on her way to becoming a cripple.

During a vacation, however, she stumbled upon something that turned her life around. She began doing modest exercising in a swimming pool and has since developed an exercise program that is done in a pool. It has made her almost pain-free. Her exercise program, like other programs that work, must be practiced regularly or the benefits quickly vanish.

Dvera's methods were lauded by Dr. F. Dudley

Hart, one of the world's leading rheumatologists. Dvera is in her mid-70s as I write this, and is an effervescent example of what a person *can* do by adapting exercise to certain physical limitations.

Consult your doctor if you suffer from arthritis, and explore the possibilities of beginning an exercise program in a pool. The buoyancy provided by the water will be a great help in alleviating some of the pain and with some careful attention to your program, you may well achieve the tremendous progress that Dvera Berson did!

There is another group of people for whom I have the utmost respect. And that is the wheelchair athletes.

During the 1970s, some courageous young men who were confined to wheelchairs found that they didn't want to be sitting on the sidelines while the rest of their friends were out running marathons. Several of these young men, some Vietnam veterans, some the victims of automobile and motorcycle accidents, began training diligently and began working politically to make a place for themselves on the starting line of many of the major marathons.

Their progress has been astounding! There are now wheelchair athletes of all ages competing in everything from basketball to marathons. Such as Bradley Hedrick, who is the head coach of the University of Illinois' men's and women's wheelchair basketball teams. He also coaches wheelchair football, and track and field. He was the first American (fourth overall) in the World Wheelchair Games marathon in England. He was also a member of the United States Olympic wheelchair basketball team. He participates in the following sports: swimming, wheelchair track and field, tennis,

softball, football, and road racing.

The wheelchair athletes have pushed the science of wheelchair manufacture forward, also. There are now all types of lighter, stronger wheelchairs available for disabled folks who are tired of being *confined* to their chairs.

It is easier now than ever for a person in a wheelchair to exercise. The same general benefits that a person receives from a regular vigorous walking program can be obtained by a person in a wheelchair who takes control of his or her own life, who gets out there and puts in miles "walking" in the wheelchair.

Your limitations are not defined by the world around you. Each person defines his or her own limitations. But, at the other end of the scale, each person defines his or her own outer limits, too.

A "walking" program adapted to wheelchair-ridden people can serve not only to promote better physical health, but can also provide incredible advances in mental health and can completely reverse one's outlook on life.

Sane, regular aerobic exercise is available to virtually anyone on earth, even the blind.

Such as Laura Oftedahl. She directs fund-raising and is public relations director for Ski for Light, Inc. This organization has been teaching blind and visually impaired people to cross-country ski since 1975. Laura has been visually impaired all her life. She runs, skiis, and bikes with a group of sighted sports enthusiasts, and has four gold and two silver medals for the United States Ski Association national disabled championships. She is listed in *Who's Who of American Women*, and her motto is, "If I can do this, I can do anything."

I couldn't have put it better.

Chapter 13

Beyond Walking

"Before supper walk a little; after supper do the same."

—Erasmus

Walking for fitness and health makes your body more able to live life to the fullest.

The feeling of being able to do more physically than you've done in years is like being reborn. It's like putting money in the bank: you build up your health account. It adds a new glow to living life.

By becoming fit through walking and maintaining your program as the framework, there are a number of opportunities open to you that allow further development of your new-found energies:

Hiking In the introduction to this book, I told the story of how I agreed to go on a hike in Yosemite with Jack not long after I first met him. As you'll recall, I got myself into a lot of trouble because I was afraid to admit to him that I was not in the best of condition. But in my mind I *thought* I was. I ended up exhausted, sore all over, and Jack wound up carrying me.

Since that day back in the 1950s, though, I've thoroughly enjoyed hiking because by getting into condition, I can do it more easily. Consequently, I now look forward to it.

Hiking can be a wonderful way of exploring the world around you, while it also provides the opportunity to see life close up and to rediscover just how wonderful nature is. A good hike through a beautiful forest can provide a rejuvenating effect. While the body gets its exercise, the mind can also exercise itself by taking in all that there is to see,

while your emotional side can just simply relax.

A hike can be as short as a half-hour. Hiking does not have to be continuous exercise like a vigorous walk should be. It can be a series of starts and stops. A good hiker is always a good walker first. Being able to walk well puts you in charge of the hike and doesn't put you at the mercy of the hike, like my Yosemite experience did to me.

Hiking provides both a wonderful physical as well as a psychological change. For more information, contact the American Hiking Society, 1701 18th Street NW, Washington, DC 20009.

Backpacking Hiking taken one giant step farther becomes backpacking. Backpacking is the process of taking along with you what you need to survive out in the woods. Certainly much more complex than hiking, you have to pack sleeping bags, a tent, cooking utensils, food (usually freeze-dried), and other equipment all neatly (well-distributed weightwise) tied up on a backpacking frame.

Whenever contemplating going backpacking, I suggest you don't lay out a great deal of money. Borrow or rent the necessary equipment in case you don't really care for sleeping under the stars. Also schedule a short (one or two nights) trip with friends who are experienced at backpacking to help teach you the ropes. Having a friend along who knows the ropes can make the difference between the backpacking trip succeeding or bombing.

Only after going on one or more one or two night trips should you attempt more ambitious expeditions. Once you've got it down, though, you'll find that backpacking is a quantum leap beyond hiking. If you want peace and quiet and unblemished wilderness, this is the way to do it. And your vigorous walking program will have placed backpacking quite within your reach.

Race-walking If you feel you have a talent for walking fast, you might want to explore the world of race walking. Don't just feel, however, that because you can make your legs go fast that you're ready for race walking. Race walking as a sport involves a very strict technique, and requires quite a bit of practice. For more information on this rather interesting Olympic sport, contact either the Walkers Club of America (445 East 86th Street, New York, NY 10028) or The Athletic Congress (P.O. Box 120, Indianapolis, IN 46206).

Jogging/Running The most logical next large step from walking is into jogging or running, a sport that has a tremendously sophisticated support system throughout the world. In many instances the walking has served to strengthen joints and ligaments and muscles, and the transition from one aerobic sport to the other is simple.

Although some people remain relatively safe from injury while walking, the transition to jogging and/or running can sometimes be a traumatic one for the joints and the bones. So if you feel that your biomechanical style is not suited to jogging and/or running, it would be best to stay with vigorous, fitness walking (Dynastriding).

If you feel you can safely make the transition, you may want to think about alternating your walking and your running, either during your run or by alternating days for running and walking. However, do so on surfaces that are going to be easy on your legs, ankles, and feet.

There are plenty of good books about running and it would be wise to read one or two before taking it up. If you need more information, contact the T.A.C. (address listed under race walking).

Other aerobic activities Once you are a good walker and your aerobic fitness level has been elevated, you will be able to expand into the much wider field of aerobic sports in general. Your aerobic fitness from Dynastriding will make it possible to take up cycling, cross-country skiing, swimming and triathloning among others. That's the wonderful thing about aerobic fitness: it translates into so many other sports. There are certain new skills to be learned, of course, such as cross-country skiing techniques, proper shifting of gears in bicycling, maximizing transitions in triathloning, etc., but your basic endurance will already be established by your walking program.

The old saying that the world is your oyster is certainly true as it applies to the aerobic oyster. Once you are fit aerobically, a whole new and wonderful world of adventures awaits you.

In short, a fit, healthy body with plenty of endurance opens a whole new world of possibilities. And it's a world where age is no drawback.

Best of luck to you as you go Dynastriding through your brave new aerobic world!

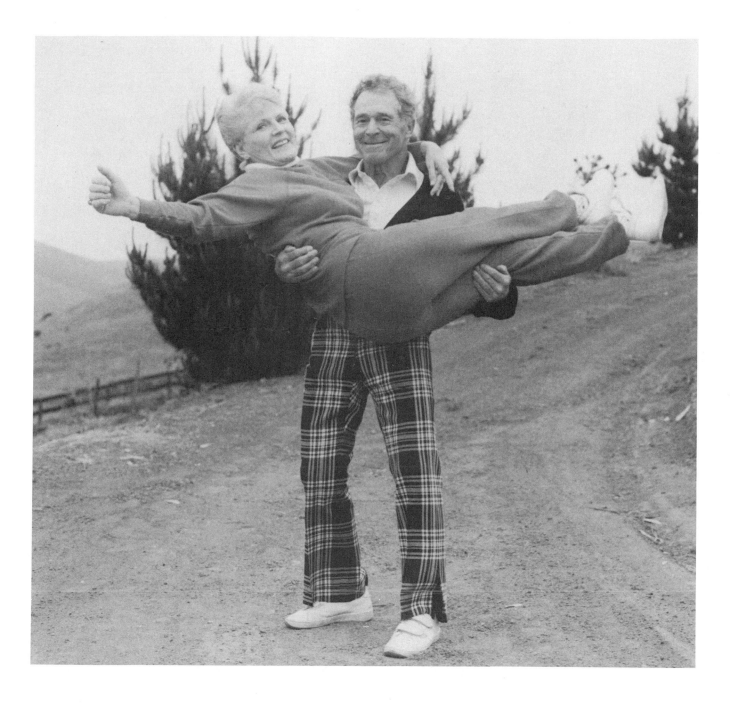